# Secrets of Plantation House


## By

## Lola Neeley

ISBN: 1-4107-3422-6 (e-book)
ISBN: 1-4107-3421-8 (Paperback)

Library of Congress Control Number: 2003092196


This book is printed on acid free paper.


Printed in the United States of America
Bloomington, IN

1stBooks – rev. 04/15/03

This book is dedicated to my three daughters, Carolyn, Lacquanna and Victoria and to the memory of my beloved son Billy Earl.

# PREFACE

Laura Dupea follows her husband Francious into a secret passage at Plantation House. There she rescues her husbands near dead grandfather from his solitary prison of seven years. Starved, emaciated his clothes rotting off his filthy body he was unable to stand alone.

Many years later someone murdered a beloved house servant, leaving her tied and clubbed to death in the basement.

In the early 1900s Willow, the sole living descendant of Laura Dupea is horribly crippled in an accident and forced to stay in her rooms for years. A fine surgeon was encountered that repaired her old broken bones and twisted muscles.

Gracie Goode, the daughter of Willow's adopted family has a terrible secret that is unearthed seven years after her death. Waiting until she is forty eight to experience her first sexual relationship, she finds the need to torture and maim her lover to reach the orgasmic peak she must have.

# CHAPTER 1

The driver called, "Whoa!" stopping the twelve seated wagon. The side flaps were rolled up to the very top of the conveyance since it was a nice warm day.

I, Nellie Farmer, stepped into the horse drawn trolley along with six excited, giggling teenage girls, all of us were headed for Plantation House where the Grover School for Girls was housed.

I personally will be housed on the third floor to see that all the girls keep to a schedule and adhere to the school rules. I will be sleeping right inside the only exit door to ensure that everyone is in bed by nine p.m. and that none left the floor until six a.m. This is the hour that everyone begins their toilette, helping each other to braid their long hair and put in the ribbons and help each other fasten their back buttons on their three quarter length dresses about mid-calf.

All the dresses are gray, high necked, three quarter sleeves with fitted tops and full skirted. All shoes are black flat heeled and have a shiny buckle across the top.

I have been told Master John's daughter Willow, is very beautiful of face but very deformed from an accident she was involved in when her mother Bess, was trying to outrun Master John as he tried to overtake her and their four year old daughter. The brougham overturned, killing Mrs. Grover and severely injuring Willow. Bones had been broken in her shoulder, left arm and her thigh. The shoulder never healed properly. The bones were never set and kept in place so they could heal straight. When Willow was seven she suffered a stroke that caused paralysis and her upper arm muscles to twist into an ugly bulge on her already deformed shoulder. Her left thigh turned outward and her left calf and foot turned inward. Still her face was beautiful and both hands were long, slender and beautifully shaped.

Willow loved music and played several instruments. Master John supplied her with everything anyone could ever need that money could buy. She had her own suite of four rooms and her combination caregiver, housekeeper, companion. A forty two year old lady that had been a teacher before she was hired as Willow's, `everything.'

Willow tried very hard to be happy and count her blessings, only…she was never allowed to leave the second floor and her father,

Master John refused to look upon her or speak to or about her. He could never look upon her or anyone or anything that was less than perfect to view.

John Grover's business (of which no one knew anything about,) kept him abroad January through October. He spent November and December at Plantation House staying in the library, which served as his office almost constantly. He came out only at mealtimes where he ate alone at the head of a fifteen foot dining table and to his bedroom in the evenings.

Each Christmas eve, Master John had all the employees line up in the magnificent ballroom where no balls were ever held. He evaluated each one according to Mora's records that she kept on personnel, as well as work abilities. He always shook hands with everyone, told them he appreciated all their efforts and gave them each envelopes containing cash. Master John was a generous employer, however he was not one to fraternize with the help or with anyone else for that matter.

Master John did not believe in using banks. He had several safes built into the walls and under the floors of closets at Plantation House.

Apart from himself only Mora knew the locations and combinations of all the safes. All household expenses were taken from the kitchen safe which was located in a false wall behind a pullout pantry shelf. All monies for the school were in the safe under the stairs and all monies for Willow's expenses were in Willow's fireplace where the mantle overlapped the stone on the right hand side. A secret latch opened the hidey hole when a certain stone was pushed three time then waited two counts and pushed it three more times fast.

Taxes, repairs, outside caretakers, supplies and so forth were paid from the safe in the library behind the shelf where law books were kept.

If something were to happen to Mora, I would become the person responsible to take over all of her duties and would have to appoint someone to take over my job should that become necessary.

Mora ran a very tight ship. Everyone was required to do exactly what Master John instructed her to have done. If one couldn't or wouldn't do their required job, they were quickly replaced.

Plantation House is huge, three stories high and each floor has ten to fifteen bedrooms. In addition to the bedrooms there are classrooms, libraries, theater rooms where the students put on plays and have music parties. All students are required to learn to play the piano, harp and piccolo. Before they graduate they will know how to cook, sew, run a house and be able to speak at least three languages, English, French and Spanish. They learn to weave and hook rugs in beautiful designs. Also prior to graduation they would be proficient in sums, spelling and the arts.

My first few weeks at Plantation House were hectic. I had to familiarize myself not only with the students and my relationship with them but with the house rules on every level.

The only time anyone on the third level is allowed in any other part of the house is at mealtime, six forty five a.m. for breakfast and five thirty p.m. for dinner. A tray of sandwiches and milk are served in the theater at noon to the students and myself. I am allowed on any floor if I make my needs known to Mora in advance.

Saturday all students are allowed to roam the grounds, lay about under the shade of a tree and in winter, play in the snow, sled, skate etc. On Sunday mornings they attend church, in the afternoon they can receive visitors, family, write letters, read or whatever else they choose to do within reason.

I first met Willow the fourth week I was at Plantation House. She is the sweetest person I have ever known. Her hair is golden with a slight reddish cast. Her long lashed eyes are green, deep green. I had seen green eyes before, but not like Willow's. Her complexion is flawless and needs no enhancement, it is like smooth white alabaster and her hands are the same. Her lips look as if they have been rouged when they hadn't, she has a small straight nose and smallish ears.

We rapidly became friends with her requesting my company whenever I have a bit of free time.

"Oh Nellie, what are the students like? Are they beautiful? Do they enjoy school or are they eager to go home?" Willow would ask me.

As I give her a rundown on the girls how old, how tall, what size family they came from she memorized their names and would demand that I bring her up to date on everyone each time I visited.

It was surprising but even with Willow's twisted arm and leg she can dance and those long slender hands moved skillfully over the piano keys and harp strings. She can make the violin sound so very sad or very happy, depending on her mood. She paints everything she can view from her windows. I am no expert but to me they look as beautiful as any of the many pieces of art that decorate the walls of Plantation House.

The longer I know Willow the closer we become. She confides her pain and unhappiness to me. "I have everything Nellie, but I'm in a beautiful prison where even my father will not visit me. I write him letters but I have never received an answer from him not even at Christmas time or even when I'm ill. I was only four when mother tried to take me and return to her parents. I am told that something about my father's business keeps him abroad and he only comes here in November and December. I remember my mother being saddened by his absences and complaining of it to him. I remember his yelling at her and hearing her cry out in pain. Later that day was when the accident happened while she was trying to leave him. Mora probably knows the truth about everything but she will never enlighten me. Sometimes I really wish that I had been killed in that accident along with my mother."

"Oh no Willow! Never even think that. You are a fine person and you have a lot to give," I told her as I held her sobbing body close to my chest.

The first time I saw Plantation House with it's beautiful cobblestone drive that curved through lovely trees and well kept grounds, I fell in love with it. Five three story columns stand across the center of the building, approximately forty feet high, gleaming white as is the rest of the house but there is a feel of something I just could not quite put a name to, like a secret doom or a hidden curse. I tried to pooh-pooh it from my mind still it lingers. Even after I was settled in I still sometimes felt the hair on the back of my neck stand out.

Mostly my charges are well behaved except small catfights break out once in awhile that I have to quieten down explaining, "Ladies do not raise their voices," or in some strong quarrels the misbehaving students will be kept in their respective rooms when the rest of the class are permitted to be outside on a Saturday or Sunday. If a student becomes quarrelsome too often, she is dismissed from the school.

The parents have to come for them and they have to face whatever punishment or scorn is meted out at home.

Always the first year is the worst time for the girls. They are homesick and not accustomed to being kept to their rooms and not having friends over other than family on the weekends. They are freed for Thanksgiving and Christmas holidays for two whole months if their family comes for them. Sadly too often some never got to go home for holidays. Their parents give excuses but the end result is rejection and tears flow. On these occasions Mora invites the girls to fraternize with the help and if they wish they can take their meals with the help as well. When Master John is home, he keeps to a strict pattern so he never encounters anyone except Mora for the accounting of all expenditures and to give instructions to.

The second year I am at Plantation House we are lined up to allow Master John to look us over, although he never makes eye contact and to accept the envelopes of cash from him. During this I notice the door on the second floor open just a crack as Willow gazed down at her father with such longing I can't control the tears running down my cheeks. Master John must think they are happy tears for his generous

9

gift. He says nothing. I spend even more time with Willow after that and a strong dislike is growing within me for her heartless father.

Mora and I often speak of Willow's pain and unhappiness and we try to think up ways to make her happier if only for short periods at a time. Mora allows select students to visit with Willow to practice music or dance. Two of the fourteen year old students are very good at art, spending much of their free time practicing at the painting of Willow's beautiful face. She won't allow any other part of her person to be painted. She, in turn paints the students, Mora and myself. At night I can hear her sobbing. Yes! I hate Master John and am happy for him to leave on December twenty eighth every year.

After Master John left for—wherever he goes, Mora gets Willow all wrapped up in warm clothing and blankets. We take Willow for long sleigh rides over the grounds. All of the students spending Christmas at school come along in sleighs pulled by shiny black horses with red decorations and bells that tinkle as we all sing Carols.

Willow is like a beautiful bird released from its cage. When we return to the house we sit around the fireplace as first one then another entertains us in one form or another. More and more Willow joins the household functions. Mora teaches her how to cook and how the house is run. She doesn't tell Willow about the safes but one day she will, after all neither Master John nor herself will live forever. Willow needs to learn how to survive on her own. Mora knows that if Master John learns that she allows and even encourages Willow to be downstairs or outside, she will be fired, however it makes no difference, she loves Willow.

The first time I help Willow bathe and dress I am almost overcome by what I know must be agonizingly painful for her. Her shoulder looks as if bones have just grown together in a jumble with just skin over them in places, no flesh. Her left arm is horribly twisted down to the elbow, but looks normal from the elbow down. The left thigh looks as though it has been broken and never set and the muscles are bunched into a twisted lump. How I kept from crying out, I'll never know. I want to ask her if a doctor had treated her after the accident but I am hesitant to upset her.

I asked Mora if Willow has ever been treated and was told in a hard cold stone voice, "No! Master John would not allow anyone to even see Willow. He let her suffer and I believed he hoped she would die. Master John always seemed to hate Willow for living while her mother had died in the crash. Miz Grover should have waited until Master John went abroad before she attempted to leave but I guess she just couldn't stand it a moment longer, he beat her you know."

I can tell Mora hates Master John as I do. Maybe he will be washed overboard at sea or get hit by a train, I hope.

Mr. Simpson, the caretaker, asked Mora if he could bring his son Daniel to help him on the grounds. Since Master John had bought up all the surrounding acreage he just couldn't keep it all up by himself. Mora knowing that no one person can possibly do all the chores on such a large place, agrees to hire Daniel.

I met Dan on the second day after he began working here. He is quite tall and muscular with dark curly hair and sparkling blue eyes and looks to be about nineteen or twenty. Dan tells me he is studying to be a surgeon and could only work part time. He still has three years of schooling to go. He had graduated high school at the age of fifteen.

Daniel comes into the kitchen to speak to Mora just as Willow is entering. She tries to back away not wanting him to see her deformity, but she trips and falls to the floor. Immediately Dan goes to her and lifts her to her feet. "Are you hurt ma'am? May I help you?"

Willow has never seen any male up close before except her father and of course Mr. Simpson. She is mortified but she sees no pity or revulsion in his wonderful eyes. Somehow she feels perfectly at ease with him.

"Yes, I could use a little help I think. It gets unhandy at times with my imperfections," she laughed.

Mora instructs Dan to carry Willow up to her room and follows close behind as he carries her with no effort to the second floor and into Willow's quarters.

"Thank you so much for your assistance. How can I repay you?" asked Willow.

"No thanks needed, but I'd like to see you again if you are agreeable. I'm studying to be a surgeon, maybe I can help you in some way."

Willow felt no embarrassment or anger. "Yes, I'd like that very much."

After Dan left Willow tells me, "Nellie, I wasn't afraid or angry or ashamed with Dan. I'm glad he's coming back."

Dan comes to me asking for details of Willow's condition. I tell him everything I have been told.

"You know it's strange but just last month we were studying a very similar case, you know of old injuries that had never been taken care of. My teacher's father, a wonderful physician was able to re-break bones and reset them. The woman is almost normal in stature now. Do you suppose Master John would allow my teacher's father to look at Willow?" asked Dan.

"Not if he knows about it, but ask Mora. She is in charge of all of us ten months of every year. Willow just celebrated her nineteenth birthday but must be twenty-one to give her own consent. I will speak to Mora. Willow is such a beautiful young woman and I hope she can be helped."

When I speak to Mora she is very nervous about allowing anyone to see Willow for any reason.

"If Master John should find out we would all be fired, then what would happen to Willow? I'll have to think on it," she said.

Time passes and it is time for Master John to return for all November and December. No one is to mention a word about anyone seeing Willow. Dan is cautioned to stay out of sight while Master John is at home.

Mora, Willow, Dan and I have decided to allow Dr. Foster to come and examine Willow just as soon as Master John leaves the last part of December. Daniel isn't taking off from school over the holidays. He is working as Dr. Foster's helper for hands on experience.

Master John has aged since his last visit, his hair is thinning and graying at the temples. His demeanor however has not changed a bit, still no eye contact, no smiles or emotion of any kind. I watched for the door to Willow's quarters to open but it did not. I am glad. Hopefully that means that Willow has accepted the fact that her father wants nothing to do with her.

We all become impatient for Master John's time at Plantation House to come to an end for ten more months. Finally he is gone. We celebrate by meeting in Willow's quarters and having cake, drinks and entertainment.

It is decided that Dr. Foster will visit in January to evaluate Willow's chances to be helped. Everyone is upbeat, hoping for a miracle. Daniel has cautioned us not to expect too much but we just can't help but hope.

Willow is so impatient to have Dr. Foster examine her and hopes he will at least be able to do something about her shoulder. Wearing long sleeves hides her arm and her dresses were all floor length to hide her thigh and foot. She told me she would just die if the doctor says he cannot help her.

Life for Willow is much happier since Mora broke the rules and has Willow join the rest of the house at meal time and is allowed to go for rides when Mr. Simpson drives one of the buggies with herself, Mora and I laughing and singing.

I do not form any relationships with any of the students that come and go from year to year. I was twenty-two when I first came to Plantation House, now I am thirty-one. All in all I enjoy my place here more than I had enjoyed my growing up years as the fourth daughter of six girls with two older brothers. Somehow I just didn't fit in as a close member of our comfortable home. Everyone expected me, as well as my sisters, to find a husband, have children and surround myself with families and their interests. I have never given much thought to a husband or to any man. I like men as friends but I do not seem to have that certain ingredient that calls for a personal relationship with anyone. I enjoy the household at Plantation House as a whole and I care for Willow because of the hurt and pain delivered not only by her injuries, but the emotional pain Master John causes her. The only real strong feeling I have ever had toward another human being is my hate for Master John. His treatment toward his daughter is unthinkably cruel.

Dr. Foster arrives on January thirteenth. He is a kindly looking and speaking man with a shock of iron gray hair, plumpish, about five foot ten and probably in his sixties. He wore a gray Hamburg hat with a gray overcoat and carried a black medical bag along with a silver headed walking stick. Smiling pleasantly, he introduces himself to Mora and she introduces each of us to him.

Mora leads him straight to Willow's quarters. After introducing Willow to Dr. Foster she says, "I'll be waiting right here when you finish Willow."

It is some two hours later that Dr. Foster reappears into the living room. Mora looks at him inquiringly. He smiled and nodded, Willow comes into the room still patting her hair in place with a big smile on her face.

"Did he tell you? Oh Mora, Dr. Foster thinks he can do quite a lot for me. I'm so thrilled," she cried.

Dr. Foster said, "I explained to Willow that I cannot treat her here. She will need to come to the clinic. It will take months just to work on the shoulder and I must have a signed permission slip to get started. I understand that you, Miz Mora, have full authority of Plantation House and those in it. Does that include Miss Willow?"

"I have been given full authority but I'm not sure Master John would agree to this or anything else that might help Willow. I'm sure Daniel has briefed you on the situation concerning Master John's attitude toward Willow. It would be necessary for Willow to be back here at Plantation House no later than October fifteenth. Master John has never arrived early but I cannot take the chance that he would and even though he never asks about Willow or visits her, someday he might."

Dr. Foster holding out a business card to Mora said, "This is my card with the address to the clinic. If you decide to do so, bring her as soon as possible."

Everyone discusses the pros and cons but we know, come what may, Willow needs to have her chance so Mr. Simpson drove me and Willow to the clinic. After getting Willow situated Dr. Foster tells us he will keep in touch with Miz Mora and that Willow can have visitors once a week in the present more often later and yes, he will have her back by October fifteenth.

"She will have to come back and she will require someone to massage and work her muscles three to four times each day. The muscles must not be allowed to stiffen up. Hot packs and liniments that I will send along must be applied. I will give instructions later."

I kiss Willow on the cheek before leaving. She looks scared and has tears in her eyes, but she is so thankful just to have a chance to be more normal and hopefully to have less pain.

This huge house and all who occupy it seem empty and lonely with Willow gone. Although we know Master John will not be turning up demanding to see Willow, we are non the less nervous and jittery. Mora had to take to her bed for two days. The pressure is just too much for her and she is turning over more and more of her responsibilities to me. Polly, one of the maids is filling in for me as housemother to the students. Everything continues to run smoothly.

Either Mora or I visit Willow each week catching up on whatever progress is being made. Willow is in great pain as the Dr. had warned her she would be for a while. Bones had to be broken and reset and twisted flesh and muscle detached and reattached in different places. In September Dr. Foster did no more surgery, saying she had to heal as much as possible to endure the trip back home. He urged her to return as soon as possible and to be very careful not to try to lift anything over three or four pounds and not to play any of her instruments. "It will probably be a year before you can chance the movement required to play," he warned.

I have learned to play the piano and the violin quite well. Now Willow and I or some of the students do duets. Of course I'm not anywhere nearly as good as Willow, but I'm happy I can play well enough not to be laughed at.

I am to have the last two weeks of December off with pay so I'm going to spend the holidays with my family. I have so many nieces and nephews I have never met and my parents are getting older. I hope we will all enjoy one another without any bickering from anyone. I know I will be barraged with questions concerning my love life, or lack thereof. I'll just have to grin and bear it.

Willow got home and feels so much better and she is so happy. She keeps looking at her shoulder in the three sided looking glass. Even with so much swelling still there, it really looks nice. I am so happy for her.

Daniel comes to check Willow's progress and to instruct us as to massage and work her muscles without causing damage to the work already done. I think Daniel has eyes for Willow and she certainly looks forward to his visits. It would be wonderful if Willow could have a happy life with someone who loves her. I pray for her.

Tuesday, Master John is expected. For the next two months the household will not be it's happy self. However we have a happy secret we keep from Master John to celebrate.

When he alights the brougham, he carries a bag of approximately eight inches thick by one and a half foot long and twenty eight inches across. He will not allow the help to carry that bag. Later Mora told me, "That's a new bag of money for the safes. There will be hundreds of thousands of dollars divided between the safes where there must be a million dollars already."

I wondered if this would mean a grater cash gift this year, as it had been three years back when he had carried that same bag into his quarters. Since I would not be there for Christmas, Mora handed me my envelope just before I left. Sure enough, there was an extra ten dollars. That was very nice but I wonder how he makes his money. Just what kind of business is Master John in and I also wonder if he has someone somewhere else that he vents his anger on as Mora tells me he did on Miz Bess, his departed wife.

Often Mora heard Miz Bess cry out and would later see bruises not only on her face but on here arms as well where the dress sleeves did not completely cover. Mora said she knew she must have been bruised over her body because every time she sat down or got up a look of pain clouded her pretty face.

"Miz Bess never confided in anyone but she was happy and outgoing the ten months he was away, treating all the help with respect. She never went anyplace and no one came to visit her. I can't imagine what Master John could find to beat her for. I could never hear his voice and he always ate alone even though Miz Bess was here," Mora informs me.

\*\*\*\*\*\*\*\*\*

## CHAPTER 2

I arrive home, or at my families home on December twentieth. The yard is full of young people and not a few dogs, all yipping and yelling at the tops of their lungs. The dogs ran and yelped and fetched sticks thrown by the children. Two sisters, Janey and Margaret along with husbands and nine children, plus my eldest brother Herman, his wife whom I had never met, with their eight children. What a madhouse. I am accustomed to order and good manners. This is mayhem!

Mother and Dad pushed through the squealing brood to embrace me and say how I had changed. I didn't point out that the years have changed them a great deal as well.

Janey hugs me and wipes at a tear on her cheek. Margaret just hugs me and pats my shoulder. By the time I have met everyone, I am overwhelmed and cannot remember which name belongs to whom. I finally got the husbands identified and Herman's wife Lolly, but I end up calling all the children, kids, or hey you!

Happy pandemonium reigns. Father takes me to look over the town comments on how it has grown. I don't recognize anyone and I used to know almost everyone around for miles. I must not have changed as much because several people called my name and waved to me.

Mother, Janey and I make pies of all kinds. Margaret made cakes of chocolate, white, spice and marble, all layer cakes. We have three turkeys, two full hams, sweet potatoes, dressing, green beans, mashed potatoes with gallons of gravy and huge salads along with coffee, tea, hot chocolate and sweet milk. Fresh fruit sits in several bowls over the sideboard and table. What a wonderful smell. I force myself not to nibble because I want to eat a washtub full at one sitting.

I am pleasantly surprised when the family doesn't try to pressure me into meeting some GREAT guy. I guess they either envy me for being free of wifely duties and running after busy children all day, or they have accepted the fact I mean to die an old maid.

I'm having a glorious time. I'm trying to recall what the reason was that I always felt like a square peg in a round hole while growing up. Perhaps it was just the fact that I felt insignificant as a fourth sister, never feeling anyone really noticed if I were there or not, or perhaps I'm just strange. I hope to be coming back every year from here on.

I must admit to being concerned as to what is going on at Plantation House. I certainly hope Master John doesn't find out about Willow being treated for anything. It's no telling what he would do. I would then have no control over my personal life if I could not find a new job that I was compatible with or capable of doing.

I know I have washed at least a thousand dishes and a ton of laundry. My hands are as puckered as a prune.

My sisters and their families have already left for their homes and Herman is leaving the same day I am. I am so happy and feel blessed to have such a wonderful family. I'm happy, happy!

On my trip back to Plantation House I met a really nice young woman and her brother Thomas. Both look to be about my age and come from a similar background, good working people religious, helpful and family oriented.

Gaylynn is a teacher and Thomas is in his last year of Veterinary school. He loves all animals and had decided to go back to school after his wife died three years ago. I liked looking at him and listened intently when he spoke. His voice made my stomach flutter. I've never felt this way before. We exchange addresses and promise each other to write, at least Gaylynn and I did. Maybe she will keep me advised as to what Thomas is up to and how he is. "Dumb!!" I scold myself, "He probably didn't even see you. He was just being friendly. POOH!!"

Master John had already departed when I returned. Everyone was in a party mood and all seemed to be happy to see me back.

"Willow! You look wonderful. Did you have a good Christmas?" I asked.

"Yes, it was nice enough I guess, but now is my Christmas. I am so glad he has left so I can breathe freely again. Look! See how my shoulder looks now and see how I can move it. Daniel said I could start using my hands more. Soon I'll be able to play again. I've really missed playing."

Everyone gathers around asking how my trip home was. As I look around at those gathered in front of me, I suddenly realized how fortunate I am to have real family. Oh yes, this family is very nice but it can't compare to blood family. However they are very dear to me and I tell them so.

Daniel comes and takes Willow back to the clinic on January second, explaining to all of us that Dr. Foster will be starting on Willow's hip and thigh next. He is leaving the work on her arm until later when the soreness would be gone from the shoulder. He also said that Willow will be in much pain again having bones re broken and reset so he wants us to keep the visits down to once a week until Willow feels as though she can enjoy company again. He explained, "All those twisted muscles have to be reattached in different locations. There is no guarantee I can make the twisted muscles work as good as new, but I can reset the bones in a more natural position and just pray the muscles will re-grow to the bones and not be so twisted."

If any serious thing happened to Willow or anyone at Plantation House while Master John was gone, none knew how to contact him. We would just have to wait until he returned. Hopefully nothing bad would happen to Willow.

I received a long letter from Gaylynn and a note from Thomas saying he had enjoyed meeting me and hoped to see me again after he finished school. I have read and reread his note trying to find something to cling to. However he did say he hoped to see me again.

Gaylynn wrote about her new students and some of the parents being too 'hoity toity' and behaving badly in front of the children. "One would think I am a servant or a poor relation to be pushed around. I'm trying to be polite and not lose my temper but I'm afraid I'm going to have to explain to these people just what my job is and what is expected of them. Oh well, time will tell."

Mora is showing me all the safes and the places where all the combinations are kept. She says I must memorize each combination. The easiest way for her to remember each one was to sing a little song like, "The safe in the hall is not very small and its numbers are, whatever they are for that particular safe. "Do it like the teachers taught you times tables, in a sing song voice."

It took me a full day at each safe to get it down to where I didn't even have to think before I quoted the correct numbers.

Mora is looking pale and she moves more slowly as time passes. She isn't really that old, maybe in her early fifties or maybe even younger. I know that she worries that Master John is going to find out we are helping Willow and that she is the one who signed the consent form. Then there is the worry of the money to pay Dr. Foster with. Master John hasn't inventoried the safes in a couple of years and it is time to do so. We were all cautioned to play dumb about everything concerning Willow. Mora is accepting all the blame.

Each time we go visit Willow she looks better and laughs a lot. She eagerly flips the sheet off to show us how straight her hip and leg is. Of course it is swollen to twice the size it was but Willow has faith. Her goal is to be able to look and walk more naturally no matter the pain. "Then," she says, "I am going to stand in line when he comes home and force him to look into my eyes. I am going to tell him what a horrible person he is and that I remember how he beat mother."

"Oh Willow, he might kill you."

"No he won't because Daniel will be there to protect me," Willow vowed. "I know I can't do it this year, but next year I can and I will."

"Willow, have you considered the fact that you will be twenty one and Master John will no longer be responsible for your livelihood?"

"What do I care? I have a trust fund left by my mother. Where do you think 'He' got his start in the first place? This house and the original grounds are mine, left to me by my mother's father and mother. All the money in the three safes in my quarters is my own. It is not money that 'He' put in there.

Even Mora hadn't known that. Willow would pay for her own surgeries with her own money. That was a great load off Mora. She had thought that he would have her arrested for stealing the funds for something he had not authorized. After that Mora perked up a little but she is still looking puny and moving at a slow pace.

The student's teacher was leaving to get married. "Mora, I know a teacher that would probably jump at the chance to teach in a private school. We met while I was on vacation and have kept in touch."

"Why don't you get a letter off to her and if she is interested, have her send me a resume along with references. We have only one month to find a replacement."

Writing Gaylynn I relayed the information Mora had imparted to me. I emphasized we have only thirty days in which to find a replacement teacher.

"Maybe Thomas will visit sometimes. I'm certainly thinking of him often. Foolish woman!!!" I thought to myself.

If Gaylynn for some reason couldn't accept or didn't want the job, I'd probably have to fill in until a replacement could be found. Oh pooh!

October fifteenth has come and Willow is back at Plantation House. Everyone is so happy to have her home. Daniel had to carry her upstairs as she clung to him it what seemed to be unnecessary closeness. I'm almost certain that Willow is smitten with Daniel and he with her.

"Oh Nellie, please come up as soon as possible. I have so many questions as well as news I want to impart to you as Dr. Foster has explained to me."

"I'll be right up Willow," I replied.

When I reached Willow's side, she was already removing her gown to show me her much improved, hip and foot. "It really does look a great deal better Willow."

"Yes, and it feels better. Of course it is still quite sore and swollen, but isn't it beautiful?" she bubbled.

The twisted muscles had been repositioned on the newly set bones in her hip and foot. It truly was a miracle. Next surgery would be done on her upper left arm to complete the reparation. If it goes as well as the rest of the surgeries have, Willow will be able to live anyway she desires.

Mora received Gaylynn's resume and references. She was eager to have the job and "Tom was happy because he could be closer to her while he was in veterinary school," Gaylynn wrote in a note to me.

Gay arrived on October thirtieth, the same day Master John arrived for his two month, stay at Plantation House. Nothing has changed with him, but I now know, or believe I know why he never allowed a Dr. to help Willow when she was injured or later when she was struck with paralysis. After finding out that Plantation House belongs to Willow and that Willow has plenty of money of her own, well, I feel that Master John had wanted her to die so he would inherit everything. Master John is a generous employer, but he seems to have a great need to be in the driver's seat, so to speak. Also I believe he likes owning things and people as well. Being generous assures him of his power to control everyone he comes into contact with. I cannot imagine his reaction when he finds out about Willow and the entire household's complicity in the act. However neither myself, nor the rest of the help would change a thing even if we could. It is so wonderful to play even a small part in helping Willow. Even with the soreness she has so much less pain than she has had to suffer before and she is so beautiful. It will take most of another year to complete the surgeries. We are all keeping our fingers crossed hoping Master John will not discover anything of the undertakings before he leaves this time. By the next time he comes home Willow, with God's help, will be healed and a whole person without pain. She will also be twenty one years of age and no longer dependent upon Master John for anything. I'm wondering if Willow will throw him out of Plantation House and take over herself, or will she let everything go along as always.

Gay is getting acquainted with her students and familiarizing herself with the house and the rules therein. She seems to like it here but has not confided in me. With Master John in residence we are all on our best behavior. I hope to be able to visit with Gay often after 'He' leaves.

Master John seems to be aging more. Each time he comes home, his hair is grayer and thinner and I've noticed this visit his stride is not as long or firm as usual. I really do not believe he is over fifty but he looks older. With his gray clothes and gray hair, he looks washed out.

I don't feel as angry with him as I did for a while. When I first heard all the stories about his mistreating his wife and his refusal to let anyone help Willow, well I just hated him. Now I just don't feel much of anything toward him.

Mora instructed me to, "Hurry up to Willow's quarters and get her into the loosest gown and robe she has and tell her not to get up or move about. Master John has informed me that he will be checking Willow's fireplace safe today. Perhaps Willow should stay in her bedroom until he has finished the inventory."

"Willow, Willow, your father is coming to check the fireplace safe today. We must get you into loose fitting clothes in the event he sees you. Hurry dear!"

"He has no right to touch my safe or anything in it!" she fumed.

"Yes, yes I know, but hold your temper. Remember you are not yet of age and you have another year before you will be healed up."

"Very well, I will hold my tongue this time. Next year I will settle with him once and for all!"

We have just finished getting Willow dressed and seated in her chair by the window in her bedroom when Master John and Mora entered. Gracious that was close. I'm still shaking to think what could have happened. I'll be so happy when `He' is gone again.

Master John left on December twenty eighth and we all breathed a sigh of relief.

After his departure, Mora found a letter from Master John on his desk in the library, which she read to me.

"Miz Mora, keep this letter and my attorney's card safe. I may not return next year, as I'm reasonably sure you are aware that upon Willow's twenty first, birthday she can claim Plantation House as her own. I'm also sure she will not want me around and with good reason. I gambled and I've lost. It sickens me to know that a grotesque thing like Willow will rule over my beautiful Plantation House. I have emptied the safe in the library and the one in my bedroom closet. The rest I'm leaving to Plantation House to keep her beautiful for all time since that is the only reason I married Bess. I wanted to be Master John of Plantation House and I have had that pleasure all these years. As you must have surmised, I have a second family abroad where I spend ten months of every year but nothing and no one can replace Plantation House in my heart. My wife's family, have all the money in the world and so do I. We have been very fortunate in money matters. Continue to run Plantation House as you have always done until Willow reclaims her property upon reaching her majority. If there is ever a change with Willow, should she die, you can reach me through my attorney whose card is enclosed.

Gratefully, John Grover

"My goodness Mora! Do you really believe he will not be back? Is there enough cash to carry on as usual?"

"Oh child, there is enough money to last several generations. I really do not understand why Master John would want to leave so much money to carry on Plantation House. I would never have believed it of him. He just said he might not return but I'm betting he does."

Mora hands me the letter to show it to Willow telling me to bring it back to her so she could put it in the kitchen safe behind the pantry shelves.

After Willow read the letter she sat very still, tears filling her eyes. "I wanted to show him how beautiful I will be on his next visit. I wonder if I have half sisters or brothers and if so does he love them and treat them well?" Slumping over in her chair she sobbed her heart out. "Why? Why?" she cried. "Why didn't he love me or even want me to survive? Why did he beat my mother? Why? Nellie I'm going to write him a letter and I want it sent to his attorney to forward on to him. I'm going to insist that he return at least this next November and face me and give me answers to all my questions. I'm going to tell him that I have a big surprise for him and I'm sending him the portrait I painted of him. He needs to know that I never gave into pain or used it as an excuse to slip into self pity."

Willow was good to her word. She also sent him a painting she had done of Plantation House.

Daniel came for Willow on January fourth. She looks so happy and hopeful. I feel very sorry for the pain I know she will have to endure. Even strength and bravery won't stop the pain.

Willow has instructed Mora to loosen the reins somewhat to allow the students more time outside for croquet and other games when they kept all their homework up. She said to have Simpson and Gaylynn drive the girls into town twice a month if they behave well. "Young people need to have some interests outside of the schoolrooms," she ordered.

When we visited Willow, we could tell she was in a great deal of pain and could hardly keep from crying out sometimes. She asked us to wait for two weeks before we visited again. She was just in too much pain for now.

Thomas came to visit Gaylynn one weekend. I was as excited as a teenager with her first date. Even if he came only to see his sister and may not even speak to me, I still hope to get a peek of him. When I saw him coming down the stairs talking to Gay, I nearly faint. He is so handsome and he has those wide, well muscled shoulders and those sparkling blue eyes.

When he sees me he held up his hand and said, "Miss Nellie, isn't it? It's so nice to see you again," as he offered his right hand to me clasping my hand in his firm grip. I tingle all over, stumbling over words of welcome to him.

"Nellie, do you have some time to walk with us? We thought some fresh air would be pleasant," she invited.

I asked Mora, "May I join Gay and her brother for a walk".

"Of course," she replied, "Have a nice visit."

Thomas situated himself to my right placing me between the two of them. I'm feeling excited. We talked about Master John saying he may not return and wondering if that were going to change anything drastically.

"Is Willow capable of running Plantation House? Will there still be the school? What ideas does anyone have that might improve plantation House?"

Thomas had moved closer to my side causing our shoulders and arms to touch once in a while. My whole body burns each time contact is made. I am afraid to look into Tom's eyes. I knew he would see the truth in my eyes. "Please," I prayed silently. "Let him care for me?" I couldn't concentrate on what Gay was saying but I heard every word Tom said.

Gaylynn said she needed to get back to her students. "All right," I said. Tom took my hand and asked if I could continue our walk a bit longer. I looked toward Gaylynn but she already had her back to me as she marched up the path to the backdoor.

"Yes, I have some free time. Where would you like to explore now?"

"Umm, how about down by the corral to look at the horses?" he said.

He still held my hand and I still felt as if I may faint. I took long breaths and tried to look composed.

When we reached the corral we were no longer in sight of the house. Tom stopped and turned toward me, his lips touched my forehead and he drew me close to his body. I didn't know what to say or do. I've never had a boyfriend and no man has ever held me or kissed me. I don't know how to kiss. I don't know if I am supposed to allow him to hold me and kiss me. However as his mouth claimed mine I am beyond reason as I cling to him trembling so badly that I will surely fall if Tom lets go of me.

"I knew the first moment I saw you that I was in love with you. How do you feel about me?" asked Tom.

"I, I don't know what I'm feeling," I stammered. "I've never been kissed before, never had a date, really have never thought about dating. However I've certainly spent a lot of time thinking about you since I first met you."

"Are you sincerely telling me you have never dated, never had a beau and have never been kissed?" Tom exclaimed.

"Yes, that is what I'm saying. I have never even considered marriage until I met you. I mean_I'm so confused. I don't know how I am supposed to behave," I cried.

"Just come here little darlin'. I'll take care of you. It just seems impossible that a beautiful lady like you has no experience. You are made for love."

We walked and talked until it was almost dinnertime and I had to go in to help in the kitchen and take food to the students. They would be served dinner this evening by their housemother. I hated to let go of Tom's hand wondering when he would be back again but I did not dare ask.

"Nellie, could you get off next Saturday? Maybe we could go on a picnic?" asked Tom.

"I'll check with Mora and be right back to let you know."

Mora gave permission so I had my first date coming up. The week flew by though I had been sure it would drag. Tom came for me in a hired rig of shiny black with yellow wheels, pulled by two equally shiny black horses. I saw the large picnic basket and could smell the fried chicken and something spicy, "Probably eggnog," I thought.

Tom put his arm across my shoulders and drove with one hand. He handled the horses with ease.

I was wondering about Tom's deceased wife. Had they been in love? Had they been happy? He must have sensed my thoughts because he began to speak about his life with his wife, whom he had been totally in love with. They both were young, healthy and content. She then died, leaving him with a broken heart and at a loss as to what he should do without her. Some time later he decided to go back to school and study to become a veterinarian since he loved animals and loved working with them.

"I have only a few more months of schooling to earn my degree. I've been checking out the need for a vet around here since Gay and now you are in this area," he smiled.

I just sat quietly beside him too tongue tied to say anything. This dating thing is frightening. I just don't know what is expected of me. I have never been shy or afraid to speak my mind. This however is different.

"How about your life up to now? Why haven't you been interested in dating, romance, marriage and a family?"

"Well, I don't really know. I was raised in a nice family of seven children. My parents are good people. They work hard and set a good example for us to follow. Somehow I just never found the idea of boys interesting. I was not interested in having the same type of family life my parents or my siblings enjoyed. I didn't go to the dances, parties or other functions the rest of my family enjoyed. I liked to read and do crafts. I liked to take long walks and I sang with the church choir. I was totally content but the family kept urging me to find a beau, get married and have babies. I just decided to find work away from family so I applied here, answering an ad in the newspaper. I've been here since I was twenty two. I've been happy and content and have become involved in Willow's illness along with the rest of the downstairs employees. Now Willow is on her way to recovery and Master John has said he would not return to Plantation House, but I believe things will remain much the same as they have."

"Nellie, do you think you could care for me and consider marriage. I mean after I have finished school and get started at a job somewhere close by. You could continue to work days here at Plantation House if Mora would consider it."

"Tom, it's too soon. I need time to figure things out. I am all aflutter with feelings and ideas I've never felt before. I'm afraid I might not be what you need, what you could be happy with."

"Fine! We have months to work things out but I can tell you right now, I love you and I intend to make you my wife."

45

There were long deep kisses making me feel as though I needed to be crushed into him. Tremors flooded my body in places I had never felt before. I wanted Tom to touch my breasts and to rub his hands all over my body. I had to control myself to keep from placing his hands on my most private parts where thrill after thrill raced with no seeming end. I was panting and trying to get all of his mouth into my mouth. My tongue of it's own accord, was darting into his mouth making him gasp.

"Wait, wait," he moaned. We must stop before it is too late Nellie."

"Too late for what?" I groaned, still trying to melt and run inside him.

Tom took my arms from around his neck and tore his lips from mine, leaving me weak and needing something more, lots more. "Sweetheart," he gasped,

"We are going to have to stay amongst other people from here on. I just won't be able to control myself and that wouldn't be fair to you. You have no experience of any kind. I just cannot take advantage of you."

"What do you mean? Did I do something wrong?"

"Oh no, you did everything right if we were already married, but as it is I just cannot take advantage of you."

"Oh but I have all kinds of urges that I have never had before."

"I know you do but we must not give into our urges before marriage."

"I just don't think I can stand not touching you Tom."

"I will be having the same feelings you have and it will be hell for me."

"Why must we wait until you finish school before we marry? We could get married and keep it a secret. I could continue working at Plantation House and we could meet sometimes to kiss and touch. Couldn't we do that Tom?"

"Oh sweet baby! I would certainly like to. Let me check into how to accomplish the fete." Again he kissed me, again I was on fire and so was he but he put me away from him and drove quickly back to Plantation House. Long after Tom was gone I was still longing for his lips, his hands. I felt like a crazy person. I wanted to run to him, stay with him forever, marriage or not. I confided in Mora asking for advice.

"Nellie, I'm an old maid, but I once had a great love that I let slip away. I've never been happy since he rode away. A year later he married a nice girl and had a fine family. Marry him as soon as possible is my best advice to you."

Two weeks later Tom and I were married by the preacher of a small church about thirty miles from Plantation House. The wonder, the beauty, the river of our love was so great we could hardly tear our bodies apart for a moment. When I think of all those barren years I missed I am astounded. Tom says never has he felt the love and the passion we share. He said he loved his first wife but it wasn't the same, not even close.

All week I wait for Saturday and Sunday so I can be back in my husband's arms. Mora lets me take off work from Friday evening until Sunday night to be with my Tom. She is happy for us and keeps our secret.

Willow came home October twentieth. She is doing really well. There is no twisted flesh and she walks normally even with the swelling still apparent. Of course there are scars, but not real bad ones. Dr. Foster is very skilled at repairing external scars as well as a great, really great, bone and muscle genius. Daniel wants to be just like Dr. Foster and I know he will be.

We are waiting to see if Master John will return this year. Willow can hardly concentrate on anything else. She has a great need to stand before her father, beautiful of face and body. I'm hoping `He' shows up.

We are getting ready for Thanksgiving. Mora says this year we are having a family dinner with all the traditional foods and a party afterwards with music and dancing. Some of the students have invited friends and family. We expect to fill the ballroom. Of course Willow has sanctioned everything and is looking forward to meeting new people, male and female.

October and November passed with no sign of Master John, but on December tenth `He' arrived, as per usual. Willow spied him from her bedroom window and hurried down the stairs to line up to greet him.

Willow was the very last person in the long line. She was dressed as all the help was dressed. When Master John came to Willow, he raised his brows looking at Mora. "We have a new girl I see."

Willow spoke up saying, "No sir, not a new girl, just a repaired girl." Looking him in the eye she slid her apron off and her already unbuttoned dress slid to the floor. She wore only a camisole and one petticoat.

Master John looked at Mora for an explanation.

"Mr. Grover, meet your daughter Willow."

Looking totally flabbergasted he tried to remember what Willow had looked like when he had last viewed her at about eight years of age. This beautiful young woman could not possibly be his child, his malformed twisted child. Willow forced his eyes to meet hers as she lifted her petticoat to show straight legs with no twisted muscles. She then turned her back to him and letting the strap to her camisole down she exposed her beautiful shoulder. Master John stared in shock and disbelief as his gaze turned to Mora for an explanation.

"A great doctor has repaired her bones and her muscles and flesh sir. It has taken three years, but as you can see she is well and happy."

"Three years! Where was she when I was here?"

"Willow came home from the clinic when you came each year. You just never bothered to visit her."

"Father, you are the cruelest person I have ever known or even heard of. You let me suffer for all those years without hope of ever having any kind of life. You beat my mother and caused her death but I have beaten you and I've beaten the odds. Plantation House is mine as well as everything in it. I accept your gift of the contents of the safes as my due for the suffering you have caused me. You may take your personal belongings and whatever you have in the library. Oh yes, the combinations of all the safes have been changed in case you have changed your mind regarding your 'gift.' Plantation House will stand for many generations Father and without any input from you."

Master John looked at Willow with sadness in his face and tears in his eyes. "I deserve any punishment you deal me. I can only apologize most humbly. I had come home to die wanting to be buried here in my beloved land. I will be on my way. There is nothing I need. I hope you can forgive me one day."

"Die? You are going to die soon? From what?" Willow demanded.

"The doctors say I have an incurable illness and can possibly last six months, or a little more," he sighed.

"Do I have any half brothers or sisters from your present marriage?" she asked.

"No, I have no children except you. I'm happy you are strong of will and capable in spite of me. I hope you will always be happy."

Master John turned to leave—"Wait, wait," Willow cried. "You do not have to leave Plantation House. Stay with us for as long as you have. Stay where you will be happy and content. We will bury you here when your time comes." Willow looked at each of us and said, "Let us all forgive Master John and make him as comfortable as possible." We all applauded and nodded our heads yes.

Willow spent every waking moment with her father. They had long talks and Willow entertained him with her music. I see her touch her cheek to his from time to time and she combs his thin gray hair.

Daniel and Dr. Foster came to meet Master John and explained how they were able to help Willow and what a brave young woman she is.

"Yes, Willow is an extraordinary human. She is very like her mother and her grandmother. They were wonderful women as well."

Willow and her father walked the land surrounding Plantation House as long as he could manage it. After he could no longer walk it, Simpson drove them over every foot of every acre. They had almost five months to become reacquainted and to rid themselves of the pain and anger they had suffered. Willow sat beside his bed holding his hand when he became too weak to be up. When he passed away Willow was devastated for weeks. She goes to his grave every day to place a fresh flower on it.

I had expected Daniel and Willow to at least date but they didn't. Willow wants to meet a lot of men before she decides on one and Daniel is taking extended courses in surgery.

On Halloween Willow gave a costume party and invited as many single men as we could locate along with many single ladies. She insisted we have twenty more males than females, giving her a chance to flirt with them all, as there would not be enough ladies to go around. The party was a huge success. Willow got all of the attention she needed. After all she is beautiful as well as very wealthy. She quickly culled out many of the young men in her mind finding them shallow and or fortune hunters. Willow has a good head on her shoulders and isn't easy to fool.

At Christmas we had another party, not inviting the fellows she had discarded in her mind from the Halloween party.

The ballroom was decorated with holly, mistletoe, cedar bows with popcorn streamers, crepe paper chains and bells made of crepe paper. Willow found an orchestra that played beautifully. We had no tree because, candles on a tree was too dangerous, Willow decided.

Again Willow conversed with, danced with and inspected the men. Again she decided on whom not to invite or date in the future. She dated pretty often but could find no one she felt she could enjoy any lasting relationship with. One by one she dropped them with only a half dozen still in the running. There was one handsome, quiet young man who was studying to be an architect that rather stood out. He didn't pursue Willow as did some of the others, but he showed up sometimes on Sunday for the croquet games and usually won. Unlike some of the other men, he did not just let Willow win to gain her favor from her. When she won with him playing, she did so fairly.

On cold days chess, checkers and bridge tables are set up in Willow's quarters. Sometimes she will play for her guests or paint them. Willow is a good hostess. No party or gathering of one or one hundred is ever dull.

"Nellie, which in your opinion is the best choice of all the fellows who come here?"

"Oh Willow, I wouldn't know that. Only you know how you feel around any or all of them."

"Well I think Wade is more sincere and we have many things in common."

"Is Wade the quiet young man that beats you at chess as well as croquet?"

"Yes he is. I feel very safe around him and I feel he is truthful."

"Has he attempted to kiss you yet?"

"No he hasn't but I haven't given him a sign that I might allow him a kiss. I'm going to though, very soon."

Wade had come to Plantation House on Saturday instead of Sunday. He knew that Willow entertained inside on cloudy days, also most visitors came on Sunday after church and he never had a chance to be alone with Willow. "I'd like to get to know her better," he explained to me. "You know like what her hobbies are, what does she intend to do with the rest of her life, what books does she like and so on?"

I went upstairs and asked Willow if she was accepting any visitors, "like Wade for instance?" I said smiling.

She said to tell him to come up in five minutes. Wade looked very happy, especially when Willow told me, "I'm not receiving any other visitors today.

\*\*\*\*\*\*\*\*\*

# CHAPTER 3

After our second anniversary, Thomas and I spent the Christmas holiday with my family with him getting acquainted and me getting reacquainted with them. Several babies have been added to the number of my nieces and nephews. I love to cuddle the babies. Everyone is urging us to have a baby even though I am past the accepted age to start a new family.

"Listen dear people, we are not doing anything to keep me from getting with child. It just isn't happening." Right away I was given all kinds of advice on how to conceive. It involved everything from drinking strong black coffee or tea just prior to making love to resting my buttocks on two pillows for at least thirty minutes after making love.

For Christmas dinner father placed two young shoats in their buried brick oven pit which had been prepared with coals overnight to heat the brick and furnish a bed for the swine to be placed on a grate just above the coals. After being seasoned and wrapped in large wet leaves, a grate was placed across the hogs and hot bricks were put on the rack before the whole thing was covered and let stand overnight. Of course we also had turkey and everything from chestnut and sage dressing to pumpkin pie as well as varied fruit and cream offerings. I have never seen so much food in one place before. At Plantation House we have huge meals daily but not like this and certainly not with all these young children and babies yelling happily.

Everyone took to Tom and he to them. Hundreds of questions were hurled at him not only about things connected to being a veterinarian, but how on earth did he get me to marry him?

Tom just smiled and winked and told everyone it was I that was looking for a husband and he just happened to be handy. Everyone laughed.

Mother was the only one not questioning me about what had changed my mind about marriage. She knew I had just been coasting and when the right one came around, "Well that's all she wrote," as the old saying goes.

Back at Plantation House there was big trouble. Mora has come up missing. Every hired hand and neighbors has been searching for her for two days. No one had noticed anything suspicious. The household is all at odds, not having anyone in charge. I got everything organized and everyone calmed down at least for the time being. Tom is staying to help in anyway he can.

Willow is put to bed crying. Mora had been her only mother figure since she was four years old.

Drinks and sandwiches are set up to nourish the searchers. The sheriff and deputies are in charge of the search.

I remember to check the pantry safe and it is empty. I quickly got my coat after checking the safes in the rest of the house. They have not been touched. I ran to some of the searchers and ask for the sheriff or a deputy. I located Tom and told him of the theft and the droplets of blood on the pantry floor. Now I am very worried. Who knows about the safe and what has happened to Mora? "Please God, protect Mora. She is such a good person."

I notice what looks like droplets of blood dotting the walk that led to the basement door. I was afraid to go down the steps so I sent one of the kitchen help to fetch the sheriff. I have carefully avoided the blood trail, not wanting to disturb any kind evidence. The sheriff examined the spots and agreed it was blood.

While two deputies held their guns at the ready, the sheriff proceeds down the basement steps holding a candle in his left hand and his gun in the right. An oil lantern is hung on a post just to the right of the last step. Sheriff Bob quickly lit it so he could see much of the interior of the basement. Mora lay in a heap in a pool of blood. Her hands are tied behind her back and bruises cover her face and arms. A long piece of wood covered with blood lay just to her left. Mora's hair is covered with blood and stuck to her head. It is obvious someone has beaten and tortured her making her tell the location and combination of the safe.

"What will I tell Willow? She loves Mora more than anyone else in the world. Who could have done such a thing and why did he take only the contents of the pantry shelves safe? I'll just bet he wasn't aware there were any other safes and Mora didn't tell. Oh Mora, why didn't you just give it to him? Probably she knew her assailant and he would have killed her anyway. Damn! Damn!"

Why hadn't the sheriff or anyone else noticed the blood droplets right at the beginning? If I can see them, so can others—however no one else knew about the safe so had no reason to investigate after glancing into the room to see if Mora was there and evidently no one had searched the basement. I'm sure it was such a madhouse before the sheriff was informed and they had told him they had already searched the house from top to bottom. The sheriff had searched her room for any kind of disturbance but had found nothing. The rest of their search had been made outside.

I wonder if Mora has any relatives and if so, where are they? I remember Mora saying to me, "Nellie, when I die, should I still be employed here, please bury me in the family area of Plantation House cemetery. This is all the family I've had for forty years." I wonder about before she started here and if she did have family elsewhere why hadn't she kept in touch with them?

My head is whirling and my nerves are frazzled. I worry for Willow as well as everyone connected with Plantation House. Will the murderer return to torture and murder me or Willow or anyone else living here?

Willow and myself are the only ones who have knowledge of the other safes. There had been well over one hundred thousand dollars in the pantry safe so maybe he won't think there are other safes here.

The safe in the library holds the most cash as well as all the important papers on Plantation House and it's occupants. I believe I'll transfer most of the cash into one of the safes in Willow's room if it is agreeable to her. I will leave about fifty thousand dollars cash in the safe since the library, to me, seems a likely place to have a safe. Should a robber ever come again, I will finally agree to show him the safe and even hand him the contents.

When we decided to tell Willow of what had happened, I prepared a small amount of laudanum to quieten her nerves and let her sleep for a while.

"Oh Nellie, have they found Mora? Is she all right?" Willow pleaded.

"Umm, first lets take this medicine and get you ready for bed."

"I've been in bed all day. I want to see Mora and I want to see her now," she ordered.

I handed her the medicine and said, "Yes, yes, but first things first." I wait for fifteen minutes before I fill her in on all the terrible details. Willow stares dry eyed, not saying a word. She then turned her face toward the wall and pulled the cover up over her head. Soon the sleep potion did it's work but Willow jerked and mumbled as she slept.

Tom has left to go back to his work and I fall into bed with nightmares of blood and torture.

When I awake the house is quiet after the noise of the searchers being here for two days and nights. I feel all poured out, like my mind and body is sedated. I'm moving in slow motion as I pour myself a cup of strong coffee which I drink as Minnie prepares a tray for Willow. Looking up I see a puffy eyed Willow entering the kitchen and becomes seated across the huge table where the help dines morning and evening.

Minnie looked at me and at the tray, "Just set in on the table please. Willow would you care for some breakfast, the tray or something else?" I asked.

"Just coffee and I would like to speak to you in my quarters when you finish your coffee. I believe we have some very important things to attend to," she stated.

"I'm ready if you are. I can take my coffee with me. We both stand each taking our coffee with us.

"Nellie I'm worried that something like this may happen again. I'm wondering what can be done to minimize the danger. Do you have some suggestions?"

"Yes, I've given it a great deal of thought and I was going to ask you how you felt about removing most of the cash from the library to one of your safes. We could leave maybe fifty thousand dollars and some of the legal papers in the safe there to make it appear to be the only safe in the household. Another thing, never let anyone know there is safe of any kind other than the library."

"I believe that is a good idea. Does Tom know of the safes?"

"No, no, I would never tell another soul in the world and if you should marry you should not share the knowledge of the safes with your husband. Plantation House will be here, many generations after we and our children's, children's, children are buried. The cash in those safes will keep it going almost indefinitely if the knowledge and whereabouts of the safes are known only to a very select person and passed to the same kind of person from generation to generation. Monies derived from the plantation itself will more than cover yearly cash to run it."

"I feel as though my very soul has been ripped out of me. I envision poor Mora being beaten and clubbed. I feel as though my insides are as twisted as my outer body used to be. The worst pain is of never seeing Mora again because of some lowly coward coveting the contents of the safe. Nellie how could anyone do such a thing for money, any amount of money?"

"I have no answer to give. I have asked myself this same question over and over. I've tried to picture who could it be. Is it someone who visits here, someone who pretends to be a friend? I just don't know. It is so very unthinkable that anyone we know would do such a thing, yet no stranger was seen lurking around. I'm thinking it had to be someone who no one would wonder about being on the grounds or even in the house. He could have slipped into the basement and just waited for Mora to send everyone off to bed as she locked up for the night. With so many folks around so much of the time, one tends to accept them without question. Mr. Simpson, the gardener, now has two helpers but none of them ever enter the house. You know they have their own quarters in the gardeners separate house some distance from the main house. Everyone knows Mr. Simpson and the helpers and no one has ever seen any of them anywhere near the house."

Plantation House goes on as smoothly as always, but there is an underlying uneasiness apparent in all of our faces. So far not a clue has been uncovered as to whom the guilty person may be. Willow has cut way back on parties or gatherings of any kind. She has lost her trust of people in general and that is sad. I worry that she may cut herself off from everyone except those of us who live here in the main house. She seldom invites any of the students to play music or paint. She says she cannot help but wonder if one of the students may have confided that Plantation House is occupied by females only thus giving someone the idea of overcoming helpless women.

Willow ordered three handguns and a double-barreled shotgun with lots of ammunition. She then had Simpson teach Gaylynn, herself and me to be proficient in handling, loading and shooting. Willow and I keep our firearms in our rooms. Gaylynn however cannot keep any kind of weapon in reach of a student so she leaves hers in the kitchen pantry where the safe had been. The safe has been removed from the wall, unlocked and placed on the floor of the pantry

to possibly throw off a robber, maybe even Mora's murderer.

Simpson and his helpers always keep firearms because of coyotes

in the calf pens and the chicken house. They are now always on the

alert. Hopefully we will never need to fire a gun, but if needed, we

know how. A lock that requires a key was installed in the basement

door. I carry the ring of keys in my huge apron pocket. Duplicate

keys are with Willow's papers, out of sight of prying eyes of anyone.

They are in the safe under the floorboards of her closet, covered by

the same carpet as the rest of her room.

"Nellie why don't you have your husband move in here with us?

We have plenty of stock of all kinds to keep him busy. I'll pay him a

good wage and you and he can have the quarters next to me. It has

five rooms including a small kitchen for private times with Tom. If

you have children there are two bedrooms and more available if you

should need them. You are my only friend and confidante since Mora

is no longer here. I'd feel a lot safer with a man around. Please!!"

she coaxed.

"I'll broach the subject to Tom. Personally, I'd love it but it's Tom's career so he must make the final choice. We could see each other every day instead of bi-weekly. Yes, I'd love that."

Tom came today, Friday, at just about sundown. I hadn't expected him until next week but he says he worries all the time he is away.

"Tom, what would you think of moving here to Plantation House to work for Willow? She asked me to consider it and offers a five room, living space plus a good wage to you. We could save both of our salaries for a rainy day," I urged.

"Honey I've been thinking of asking you to move into town with me but I know you love it here so I've put it off. Yes, I think my working here is a great idea. When do I start?"

"I'll take you up to Willow's quarters. You can discuss the details with her while I close up down here."

In Willow's room I said, "Willow, here is Tom. He is anxious to hear what your offer is." Closing the door I left them to their arrangements.

An hour later Tom came to my rooms. Smiling, he gathered me in his arms kissing me soundly. "Did you make a deal?"

"A wonderful deal. I'll be making twice what I do now and I can spend every night with you," he laughed.

We made love all night, wonderful love, blissful love, sweet love and happy love. Happy, happy!

I hated to roll out of bed at four thirty the following morning, but it is my weekend to manage the kitchen as well as the rest of the household. Tom sleeps away, not having to rise for two more hours at six thirty to start his first tour of the plantation and inspect the animals. I am tired but I am happy. It was so nice to have my husband in my bed and to look forward to the same every night hereafter.

Since Master John died, we have added another table to the one he always sat at alone. We can now seat all of the students and ourselves, Willow, Gaylynn and me and now Tom, instead of part of us sitting in the kitchen to eat. Today though, Willow decided to have a tray in her room.

The students blushed at seeing Tom sitting at the head of the table in Willow's absence. They had never had a male sit with them at mealtime in Plantation House. They were quieter than usual and kept their eyes on their plates. None asked for seconds as they normally did. They will soon become at ease with Tom's presence and everything will be back to normal.

When Tom came in he said, "There is a never ending stream of cattle, horses as well as smaller farm animals. I'll be hard put to tend all of them all the time. I love it. Simpson and the fellows are a fine group of men, friendly, helpful and capable. You can tell they love animals by the way they treat them. They love the work but need at least three more men since all of the added land is sowed in wheat and clover hay. Next year Simpson intends to plant alfalfa to feed the extra cattle. They have always hired extra men to bring in the crops and round up the cattle to sell. It would be better to have another three or four permanent men that know what is expected of them and know how to do it, than to depend on transient workers you don't know and have them hanging around."

"Perhaps you should speak to Willow about it."

"Right, I'll do that."

After supper Tom knocked on Willow's door. "It's Tom," he called out.

"Enter," Willow answered.

"I've been speaking with Simpson and he tells me we need three or four more permanent hands since all the added acreage has been sown with grains as well as having an extra thousand head or so of cattle. We must put on extra men at roundup time and for driving animals from pasture to pasture. Simpson says the plantation is very large and he doesn't know the exact acreage but believes it to be well over twenty thousand acres with room for another thousand head of cattle. Water is plentiful with several lakes scattered over the acreage."

"I'll think on it. Send Simpson to my quarters at eleven a.m. tomorrow please," smiled Willow.

Tom gave Simpson Willow's orders and then set to work helping the cows that were dropping calves. He was so engrossed in his work he forgot to come to the house for sandwiches and coffee at midday. His stomach began reminding him by mid afternoon. By suppertime, he said his stomach thought his throat had been cut. I piled huge amounts of food on his plate and he asked for refills. The girls laughed. They have gotten used to Tom's jokes and look forward to seeing him at mealtimes.

I have not been feeling quite up to par as of late. I may have picked up a cold. My head hurts and I tire easily. I've been overeating also. I just feel hungry but nothing seems to satisfy me. If I don't watch it I'll get as large as one of those cows Tom works with.

Willow's friend Wade, has sent a couple of notes to her asking to come and see her or to allow him to escort her to the theater next week. I don't know if she is considering going or not. She hasn't accepted any callers for months. I hate to see her shut herself off from everyone. She is just too young to stop her normal life and become a recluse. She has so much to give to some fine man and she is worthy of love. She should have children to continue Plantation House. I believe I'll broach the subject from that position. Plantation House means everything to her.

When I went into Willow's living room, she was just sitting, staring out the window. She looks as though she has not even combed her hair and she has not gotten dressed all day.

"Honey," I began, "It isn't good for you to spend so much time by yourself. How are you going to find a gentleman to father the babies you must have to pass Plantation House on to?" I laughed.

"Babies? What babies? Who can I trust to even date? How can I tell what a man is really about? Is he looking to get his hands on the plantation or deciding to rob and kill me?"

"Willow, you must stop distrusting everyone you come in contact with and you must have heirs to leave the plantation to."

"Then you pick someone out for me, I cannot choose."

"I can't do that Willow. Only you can feel the pull of your heart and your body."

"I feel nothing for any man Nellie. I'm dead inside and I probably couldn't have children anyway. You have the babies and I'll will the whole plantation to you and yours."

"You don't mean that honey and besides I haven't been able to get pregnant yet. Maybe I never will."

"I must have a long lost relative someplace," Willow said. "Lets start looking through all of the records in the safes. Maybe there is some cousin who has a dozen children and is just hoping for a miracle."

We have searched through every safe and looked at all the bible's entries where families are listed for generations. However not one name is listed except for Willow's, her parents and her grandparents on her mother's side. Master John had no listing for anyone on his side of the family.

"Well, I know darned well father wasn't just hatched. He had a mother someplace. Lets contact that lawyer of his," she spat.

The letter and the business card was in Willow's fireplace safe where we had placed it for safekeeping. Willow sent off a letter to the attorney, identified herself and asked him for any information on any family members of John Grover excluding his wife or her family who lived abroad someplace.

Two months later, Willow received a letter from the attorney. He said he had been unable to locate any information on the birthplace or birth date on John Grover or any family members other than those of his wife at the time of his death.

I'm still feeling headachy and tired and sure enough I've gained weight. My skirts are tight and make me uncomfortable and my feet swell.

Tom noticed my weight gain and teased me about my eating all the time.

"I can't help it. I feel a gnawing in the pit of my stomach all of the time and if I don't eat something, I feel queasy."

Tom looked at me for a moment then smiled. "Betcha you are pregnant." Picking me up and kissing me he then grabbed his back acting as though he had broken it from lifting me.

"Oh stop it. It isn't that bad!" I pouted.

"I'm just playing but you do need to see a doctor," Tom said.

I did and sure enough, I'm four months pregnant. After telling Tom I rushed in to tell Willow. Her face lit up with a lovely smile that I had not seen in quite a while. She sat right down and began to write her will leaving everything to me and my children and their children and so on. Tom was to receive all the stock on the plantation and a regular annuity for his lifetime. We did not tell Tom. No one was to know until after Willow's death, which I hoped was a very long time off.

I gained a lot of weight and continued to feel famished. I'm about three weeks from my delivery date and have to be pulled up off chairs and the bed. I have turned my job over to Minnie until after the baby is born and probably for a couple of months after that.

Minnie has proven to be a good solid employee. She works hard and is intelligent. The rest of the household like and get along well with her. No one seems to resent her being chosen as my second in command. She and Timothy, one of Simpson's first two helpers are going steady. Timmy is a fine young man according to Tom and Simpson.

I awake at one a.m. with a terrible backache and cramps. I wake Tom and he immediately sent Timmy to fetch the doctor. By the time the doctor arrives I am yelling my head off. My entire back is in spasms and I am cramping so hard and constantly I just want to die.

"Do something, help me. I can't stand this pain. I'm too old to be having a first baby," I scream.

The doctor is placing hot steaming towels to my private parts. He says it's to help keep my flesh from tearing. "I don't care what it's for, just make it stop. Oh I've got to use the chamber pot. I've got to go."

"That's all right Nellie, just go ahead," said the doctor.

"Oh no, I can't do that, I must get up," but right at that moment I have the most terrible pushing pain. I grunted and screamed and I hated everyone. "Why aren't you helping me? Tom do something," I begged.

I can see Tom's face and he looks scared to death. All at once I have another pain causing me to bear down with all my might, then I hear the baby cry. I can't see the baby or the doctor but Tom is smiling, then shock comes over his face as another baby comes out howling lustily. He, or she is howling his lungs out. For a short while I am in reasonable comfort then comes a big pushing pain and the afterbirth slides out. I don't want to see the babies. I just want to sleep. I awake about seven thirty a.m. when I feel someone putting a baby to my breast. I look down at a mass of black curly hair that tops a beautiful baby as it nuzzles trying to find the nipple, which is finally accomplished with the doctor's help.

"Well Nellie, you have fine twin boys. They are perfect," the doctor informed me.

"Really? Two healthy boys?" I cry, as one nurses eagerly. They are so beautiful. They look just like Tom. The other baby came to my breast and suckled hungrily. He is the exact image of his brother. "Tom, Tom, what are we going to name them and how can we tell them apart?"

"I don't know what to name them. I didn't expect two."

"Neither did I, but they must have names."

It is now three days later and we have still not named the twins. I think Tom has about decided on John, after Master John and Tom after himself. Their whole first names will be Jonathan and Thomas. Willow is thrilled to have Jonathan named after her father. John has one little toe that is shorter than the others and Tom's ear on his right side is shaped a little differently than his other. We wrote it in the Bible so we wouldn't forget which twin had what.

The babies are all that Willow wants to talk about or have anything to do with. She is totally wrapped up in both of them and watches over them while I am working. We have to supplement my breast milk with bottles of cow's milk. The boys are going to be whoppers if they continue to eat like they do now. Gratefully I lost my extra weight. The twins get the benefits of all my food, so I lost weight right away. They look more like Tom every day and he is so proud of them he could burst. Every time he has a free moment, he comes to check on them and to cuddle each of them. Tom is so eager for them to have a good education he saves every penny he can. I cannot tell him their future is secure or that he doesn't need to do without to ensure they have everything they need.

No information as of yet of Mora's killer. It has been nearly two years since her death.

Wade is still holding on trying to entice Willow to see him. Perhaps she will decide to after the new wears off the babies for her.

When the twins were six months old I knew I was pregnant again. I'm not really looking forward to the discomfort of the pregnancy and certainly not to the pain of birthing. However I do hope to have one

79

little girl, then no more babies. When Tom came in from work I told him that I was with child again. At first Tom looked very concerned, but soon held me on his lap and began saying girl's names.

"What if we have another boy?" I asked.

"That's all right. I'll take another boy or two," he said.

"Oh no! I'm not having twins. I can't do that again. I got so big last time I felt like a hippopotamus."

"I guess we will just have to take what we get," Tom smiled.

**\*\*\*\*\*\*\*\*\***

# CHAPTER 4

The twins are having their sixteenth birthday party today. I'm feeling very old. Gracie, my lovely daughter is going to be fifteen soon and not long after all of my children will be off to their respective schools. They will be leaving the household wishing for summer so the children will return home again.

Since Willow finally allowed Wade to come around again some ten years past, the children spend more of their time with their father learning about caring for animals.

Lately Wade seems to have something eating at him. Tom and I as well as Willow, are hard put to know what it could be.

Of course he is always pushing Willow to marry him and to stop seeing other men, which she has been doing for the past ten years. For five years or so after Mora was murdered, Willow would see no male. Little by little she began to entertain again, giving parties and having musicals in her quarters. She has also become a very well known artist, doing portraits as well as still life.

Wade has been roaming about the house, poking around and asking questions on how Plantation House is run. He asks if the cattle, grain, horses, etc. make the profit it takes to run a huge house and acreage the size of this?

Willow will never answer his inquiries and has instructed everyone on the plantation to never give out information to anyone. Not that they could. No one has privy to that kind of information except Willow and myself.

"Wade" said Willow, "I do not believe we should see one another for a while. You are out of sorts much of the time and I do not wish to deal with whatever your problem is."

Willow confided in me that Wade's eyes looked as if he could kill her, but that calm face of his remained expressionless as always.

"Honey, being around one person so much of the time can get to be a real drag. Probably some time away from him and he from you will be good for both of you," I advised her.

Willow asked me if I knew where Wade lived or how he made a living.

"Nooo, I really have no idea. At first he was in school studying architecture, I believe he said. However I've never heard anyone say anything about him having a job."

"I'm going to have someone run a check on him," Willow said. "I've never been interested enough to even question him about anything personal."

The investigator Willow hired reported to her that until six months past Wade Allen had lived in a very nice home with two servants, often giving lavish parties and handing out generous party favors. However he now resides in a rooming house in the next town south from here never seeing any of his old acquaintances. He had never been known to work and he had never finished architectural college since he had come into an inheritance from a relative some seventeen or eighteen years ago.

As Willow read the information concerning Wade's history, her voice quavered and her hands shook. She at once suspected Wade of murdering Mora and robbing the safe.

"Oh Nellie, we could have all been murdered at any time. That sneak, that horrid pretender. All these years he has been pretending to pursue me. He was actually trying to get information on Plantation House, it's acreage, how we finance it and roaming about, trying to locate safes no doubt."

"Willow, we must not let Wade or anyone else other than Tom and Simpson know anything about what we suspect until we can set a trap for Wade." I called Tom into the house and we went immediately to Willow's quarters.

Tom is in shock and so angry he wants to attack Wade at once.

"No, we must not do that. We have to have proof and we must plan carefully," I warned Tom.

"Every time I close my eyes I see Mora's battered body," Willow moaned.

The entire plantation was off limits to everyone other than employees. No one could enter the grounds and should someone slip through, we warned the employees to keep the doors locked and refuse entry to everyone.

Minnie asked, "Even Mr. Wade should he come to call?"

"No one, I repeat 'No One' is to be permitted into the house and anyone calling is to be reported at once," I ordered.

Our firearms have been cleaned and fired to make sure they are in good working order. Tom and Simpson along with Timmy and Reginald, Simpson's best help, are now strapping on their firearms every day and keeping them at their bedsides each night.

Two weeks later Willow invited half a dozen guests, Wade amongst them, to a small gathering in her quarters. We downstairs folk had an impromptu party for one of the kitchen help, which included Timmy, Reginald, Simpson and Tom. My role is to let slip that the safe in the library is faulty and we will need a repairman tomorrow. I made sure to drop this information to Willow in the presence of Wade.

"Yes Nellie, be sure to get a safe locksmith early tomorrow," Willow instructed.

An hour later Wade, holding Willow's hand, asked her to excuse him. "My head is bursting," he told her.

"Of course Wade," Willow smiled. "Come by next Saturday for games," she invited.

Tom, Simpson and the two young men are well hidden where they can see anyone entering the library. If Wade shows up, they will wait until he opens the safe and some of the contents in his hand before they grab him.

It was past two a.m. when everyone was supposedly in bed, that someone opened the library door, closed it and lit a candle, which he was holding in his left hand. Wade stood looking around trying to guess where the safe might be. I had left the framed painting slightly askew over the space the safe was hidden.

Slowly, being careful not to bump into anything. Wade approached the painting, carefully taking it down and exposing the safe. It was not locked. He reached in and withdrew the many papers and the stacks of bills. Just as he turned to leave, Tom and Simpson grabbed him.

"I just cannot help it. I have to beat the shit out of him," Tom told the other men. When Tom finished with him, Wade looked almost as bad as dear Mora had looked. Wade was tied up and held until the sheriff got there to pick him up.

Investigation into Wade's background and his interrogation by the sheriff uncovered a long history of theft and robberies. Wade had been sentenced to three years in prison when he was eighteen for robbery and assault. Upon his release, he manufactured a history of school and wealthy parents. After meeting Willow through a mutual acquaintance who had taken him to Plantation House on a Saturday, he had set about winning her. He thought that through her he would have control of the plantation and any monies she might have. He said of the robbery and the murder of Mora, "I waited in the basement until everyone had been sent off to bed, except for Mora. It had been my intention to only steal something of value that I could sell for 'getting along funds' but Mora had decided to go down into the basement to check out supplies I presume. I bumped something, she heard me then she saw me. She asked me, "What on earth are you doing down here?" I guess I looked scared or something because it seemed to startle her and she ran up the basement stairs and I caught her by her foot as she reached the top of the stairs and she fell hitting her head. She was knocked unconscious. I knew no amount of talk was going to smooth this over so I revived her and banged her around with my fists for a while. When I realized she wasn't going to tell me anything about where the safe was or any money was kept I continued beating her. I knew every large place kept household money on the premises for the running of the house at least. I picked up a long piece of wood and started beating. Still she would not say anything until I told her I would go do worse to Willow if she did not reveal the location of the money to me. Finally she gasped out that the safe was in the pantry behind the shelves. She was bleeding badly and I started to finish her off then until I remembered I would need the safe's combination. The damned old hag kept giving me the wrong numbers so I lifted her to her feet and took her to the pantry. After some more beating and more threats of what I'd do to Willow, she opened the safe for me. I took her back to the basement and tied her hands. I sat for a bit wondering what to do. Finally I realized there was no option, I had to kill her. I couldn't leave her alive to identify me as the robber, so I crushed her skull and made sure she was no longer breathing. I took all the money from the safe, something over two hundred thousand dollars. That financed me in the lifestyle I had always wanted to live. I finally had to tone down my lifestyle, but I had become accustomed to the finer things. A few months ago I knew I was going to have to convince Willow to marry me—or—well you know what happened," he sniveled.

I'm pleased to say that it took only ten days to hold court in our newly built courthouse and to hang the dirty skunk from the town's bell pole. I did not go to see the hanging. Neither did Willow nor any of the other ladies who are employed here at Plantation House. However all of the males went and yelled swear words at Wade as he was dropped through the trapdoor of the gallows. Later they celebrated by going to Slattery Alice's Saloon for a few drinks. Tom did not get home until almost midnight. I'm guessing he was trying to forget about seeing a human being die, no matter how much it was deserved.

Willow has not gone back to hibernating, as I feared she would. She is having a social gathering this Sunday after Sunday school. There will be fifty or more persons here so I must get plans underway.

\*\*\*\*\*\*\*\*\*

# CHAPTER 5

The twins and Gracie will be home tomorrow for the holidays. I am so looking forward to seeing them. I just cannot believe the twins will be twenty one in a few weeks and Gracie will be twenty her next birthday. Jonathan is bringing a friend to spend the holidays with us. I'm looking forward to meeting her.

Thomas has not confided anything of his love life, though I'm sure it won't be long until he does. Thomas is studying to be a veterinarian like his father. Jonathan is majoring in business management and intends to oversee the running of Plantation House sometime in the future. He has always been closer to Willow than Thomas is and Willow has been grooming him for overseer all of his life.

Already quarters are being readied for the boys. Gracie will stay with Tom and I until she marries or decides to go elsewhere, as I had done.

\*\*\*\*\*\*\*\*\*\*

# CHAPTER 6

Sunday, December ninth, Jonathan married his long time sweetheart, Harriet Smith. The wedding has been planned down to the tiniest detail. Both Jonathan and Harriet look beautiful and one can see the love in their faces. I'm so happy to see one son settled into marriage. I'm hoping for a grandchild the first year and many more to follow.

It was just after midnight when the storm struck. First there was heavy blowing rain that tore shutters off and beat them against the windows. Later an ice storm of gigantic proportions froze everything solid. Trees looked like crystal being whipped by the wind. The windmill froze solid. The poor animals huddle together trying to keep from freezing to death. There is no way to shelter thousands of cattle and horses over the pasture- land. For two days the storm rages and everything is frozen solid.

Minnie is due to have her and Tim's first child. No doctor can possibly make it through this freezing storm. We have prepared a birthing room with everything it takes to bring a baby and mother safely through the birthing ordeal.

Finally we can venture outside. There is nothing but ice-covered ground as far as the eye can see. Huge limbs have broken off from hundred year old trees. They litter the grounds where the weight of the ice and or wind has deposited them. The sun is shining brightly but no thawing is happening. It is so cold that the hairs in our noses freeze at once. Tom made his way to the barn to feed the animals kept there and to break the ice in the water troughs. Even under cover the animals were in bad shape.

A week later the temperature is still below zero and no change can be foreseen for days, maybe weeks. Jonathan and Tommy are very concerned for the cattle that have been in the open all this time. Tom says we will lose hundreds, maybe thousands of cattle from freezing. Some of the frozen animals will be butchered for house meat. The rest will have to be skinned for the hides and many will be buried. With that many dead, or expected dead, the carcasses will cause unhealthy conditions for the surviving animals. Tom said, "I'm afraid most will be dead before we can get to them."

The capital loss will be great, but our concern is for the poor animals. Plantation House will survive.

Tom and the rest of the men loaded wagons with hay to feed any cattle they might find alive. They took sledgehammers and axes to chop holes to water them. It is very slow progress and dangerous for the horses trying to pull the wagons and keep their footing. For miles Tom found only a few stranded cows, all frozen to death. He is surprised to have found so few cattle dead or alive. The farther they go the more surprised he feels. Where could all the cattle be? The farther south they go the more animals they find, all dead except for a dozen or so that have gone into a gully where they are somewhat protected. However they cannot get out of the gully because the ground is so frozen they cannot climb the incline out of their prison of ice. Hay and grain are put out for them. Nothing can be done about water but ice can supply them with enough water to sustain them for a while. The ice is becoming less and less the farther they go. It seems as though the storm was less severe the farther south they travel. The sun is shining and thawing is taking place. Cattle are now being found alive, some just barely. They come running to the wagon for hay and grain. The men cut holes through the ice at several of the watering holes. After unloading all the feed, they head for the house. It is getting very cold the nearer to sundown it gets. They would never be able to survive a night in the open.

Each day the men go out searching for more cattle. They unload feed and break ice trying to save as many cattle that are still alive as possible. Each time they come back to the barn, they bring one or two of the frozen cattle. They skin and butcher them until every place to can, store or cook meat is filled to capacity. As a rule they only butcher a cow twice a week to supply the house and Simpson's crew with meat. It seems as though most of the cattle migrated to the south, missing the storm at it's worst. I have always been told that all animals have a sixth sense about storms and earthquakes and will move away from certain places when there is no fence to hold them in. Maybe, just maybe, that is what has happened to our cattle.

Two weeks after the thaw begins, the men try to make a count of the dead animals, which includes over one hundred horses. As nearly as we can estimate we lost between nine hundred and a thousand animals in all. The plantation's men employees skinned most of the dead animals and took the still frozen meat into town handing it out to anyone who wanted it. We try never to waste anything if we can find use for it anywhere.

As the ground thawed and became soft again, the men dug holes, pushed the animals in and set fire to them to help protect the rest of the herd.

The mending of the damage done by the storm to Plantation House is put off until spring. It is just too cold to do it now, besides the men are loaded down with other chores all over the plantation. We are keeping the milk cows in the barn now, well fed and milked morning and evening as usual.

I am so proud of my children. They are loving, well mannered young adults. Both boys are six feet two inches tall, well built, healthy and so handsome.

Gracie is petite with natural curly hair and blue eyes, just like her dad's. Willow is instructing Gracie in music, dance and painting. We are teaching her to cook and to sew beautifully.

Jonathan and Thomas keep inviting young men to visit for Gracie to meet. However so far she hasn't shown interest in any one person.

Harriet and Jonathan are having a baby in three months. They are so happy and she hasn't suffered morning sickness or backaches and swollen ankles up to now. I hope she continues to feel well and I pray the birthing will be easy for her. She is young, much younger than I was. Surely that will make it easier on her. Tom is just as thrilled as I am, so are Gracie and Thomas.

In Harriet's eighth month, her water broke in the middle of the night. She had not had any kind of pain nor did she suffer any pain through the rest of the night. She said she was just hungry. When the doctor arrived he made an examination finding no evidence of dilation. The doctor left at about two p.m. saying to come for him if we needed him. Harriet didn't have any discomfort through month nine, until the day she was due to deliver. When the pains did start, they were severe and fast, coming one after the other causing her to cry out in agony. The doctor arrives and examines Harriet to see how far she has dilated.

"Umm, she is ready now. Everyone except Nellie and Jonathan please leave. Show my nurse in please," the doctor says. Harriet is crying out and pulling at Jonathan who tries to calm her with words of love and courage. He holds one arm around her shoulders until the doctor told his nurse to place Harriet's hands through the loops in the rope that is tied to the poster bed. He instructed Harriet to "Push!— Push hard!"

Harriet shakes her head no. "It hurts too much!" she screams.

The nurse whispers to Harriet, "If you don't push, it will last much longer. Now bear down, just like you do when you expel stool."

Sweat and tears made her pushed up gown damp. Finally after hours of pain Harriet delivered a beautiful baby girl, very red and howling loudly.

Jonathan held Harriet in his arms telling her how proud he is of her and how much he loves her. When the nurse presented their tiny wrinkled baby to them, their eyes were bright with tears of happiness.

*********

# CHAPTER 7

The years are passing quickly at Plantation House. Tom and I now have four grandchildren, all from Jonathan and Harriet, one girl and three boys. They are now nine, seven, six and two years of age.

Thomas finally married but they have not produced a child, so far.

Gracie left Plantation House to study art in Paris. We do not hear from her often. I remember when I left home not to return for years and seldom writing. I'll just have to wait until she decides for herself what she wants out of life.

Willow has done much research on the former Masters of Plantation House back to her great, great, great grandmother who inherited it from her Frenchman husband back in the 1700s. In that era it was practically unheard of for a woman to inherit property. However Francious Dupea had no male relatives to claim title to Plantation House so great, great grandmother ended up with everything. She had only two children, a boy and a girl. The son died shortly after his birth so great, great grandmother inherited. She also had only one child, a female. Willow's grandmother left everything to her only daughter Bess. Willow's mother became Mistress of Plantation House as well as inheriting extensive wealth in the form of jewels, paintings, cash and many animals. Bess had put everything in Willow's name before she was killed leaving Master John completely out of her will except that he was to run the plantation for as long as he lived. Nothing could ever be sold or mortgaged nor could it be transferred to anyone unless Willow wished to dispose of it after her twenty first birthday. Certain monies were the sole possession of Willow and not to be spent on the running of the plantation. However it was to be added to from profits gained from the sale of whatever could be grown or manufactured on the plantation.

Further, at no time were slaves to be owned or used to work the house or lands. Not many northerners owned slaves but Bess wanted to be very sure that none would be purchased by any future Masters of Plantation House.

Now there will be no blood relations to leave the plantation to. Willow is the last of her family line. Now only my children and their children and generations to come would ever own any part of Plantation House.

Jonathan feels the responsibility of running every phase and all of its endeavors, as Willow's grandmother had wanted it to be. He is raising his eldest son to take his place in the future as Master of this beautiful place, since Willow finally explained to him what she had done and has shown him her will.

I had kept the secret all these years from Tom as well as the children. Tom was somewhat hurt until I explained the necessity of secrecy while the children were young. We were worried that had they known how much they have they might not try as hard to be strong, self sufficient, people.

Tom and I no longer toil. We enjoy the grandchildren and each other along with Willow, who like us is getting along a little slower now.

Willow has never married although she dated quite a bit and had a few short relationships. She says, "I feel no shame in satisfying my physical and emotional needs. Biological urges are normal and should not be stifled.

Gracie came home when she was twenty five. Her music and art take up all of her time. I doubt if she will ever marry. However I was older than she when I met and married my Tom. She has moved in with Willow where they paint, play music and have long talks. Most of the time neither of them join the rest of us at mealtime. Willow had appointed Gracie to take over my position when I retired, which I now have. I feel confident Gracie will be a wonderful keeper of Plantation House.

\*\*\*\*\*\*\*\*\*

# CHAPTER 8

Mother and Father no longer take much interest in the management of the plantation these days, so I, `Gracie Goode' have accepted this position as keeper of the history of Plantation House, as well as the duties required to keep it running smoothly.

I miss the free time I had to pursue my music and art lessons from Willow. I also miss the time I spent with Willow. I am training a German lady to take over the running of the kitchen as well as all the first floor duties, leaving me time to enjoy my life somewhat better. Mother felt the need to have complete reign and control over every aspect of the house. I however, do not believe everyone and everything will fall apart if I am not hovering about. Hilda is a very responsible person with a strong sense of duty. She also has a way about her that allows her to get the most out of household help without making them feel resentful.

There were dark days for Plantation House when one of the students brought diphtheria into the school just after Christmas holidays. Although we segregated the students that had been exposed to the disease as quickly as possible after Cordia was diagnosed, it spread through the rest of the house, including myself. All of Plantation House was quarantined with all food and supplies prepared in the separate kitchen the outside help were fed from and carried it to the now severely understaffed house kitchen's back door to serve the household. The doctors that had already had the disease before came and went. They entered in hospital wrap around cotton robes and departed in freshly laundered clothes, which they changed into before they left. Dr. Filmore lived at Plantation House for three months. I don't know how any of us could have survived without him.

Mother and Father succumbed to the illness, as did two of my nieces and one nephew. The loss of them devastated Willow and myself, as it did the rest of the family. We also lost three servants, all females and two of the students including the girl who had originally brought the sickness to the house.

Diphtheria is a terrible illness. The throat swells shut with huge pus filled blisters that choke a person so one cannot swallow anything, not even water. High fever and general discomfort plague the entire body and sleep is impossible. In this day and time there is little that can be done except to bathe the patient and try to get liquids into them. Bloodletting is sometime used, but Dr. Filmore said that would further weaken the body and cause loss of strength to heal the patient. Even though some of the doctors that came insisted bloodletting would help, I had more faith in Dr. Filmore and refused to allow any of the other doctors to use it as a possible aide in the treatment available.

For months everyone in the house looked tired and worn. Weakness and apathy, weight loss and nervousness were evidenced.

Parents of some of the students came to take their daughters home. Some however, never even came to visit or even inquire as to the health of their children though they had all been notified of the sickness. I often feel 'Grover School for Young Ladies' is just a way for some parents to rid themselves of the responsibility of their children's daily needs. I'm always so sad when I look into a student's eyes and see that abandoned look. Their tears flow and they often stay in their rooms refusing to go to class. These girls, Willow and I try to reach through music and art as well as one on one, conversations. We spend as much time with them as possible. None of my family ever sent our children off to school. For college, they are allowed to choose where they will go and every holiday, they come home or we go to their college. Some of the female members of our family just do their schooling here at Grover. The boys however go for specialized training at colleges closest to home if possible. I'm happy I was able to travel and see so many places before I settled into life here on the plantation, but I'd never want to live anywhere else. Family and heritage is very important to me.

Soon it will be time for a family reunion. I am looking forward to meeting the many relatives I had missed meeting while I was abroad. It is always held in June after school closes for summer vacation. However the exact date has not yet been set.

\*\*\*\*\*\*\*\*\*

# CHAPTER 9

Jonathan and Thomas, the eldest of our immediate family are in charge of all outside workers and all management of the plantation. They do all the hiring and firing of the outside help it takes to run the plantations many and diversified projects.

We run thousands of head of cattle and horses and swine into the hundreds. We also have grains and hay for all the animals as well as some left over to sell. Huge gardens and a fine orchard are once again producing after the loss of so many trees in the big ice storm some years back when trees were killed due to the substantial freezing weather. We have a small herd of goats for the times when some of the babies cannot tolerate cow's milk or mother's milk. We maintain a flock of chickens to keep the house and the men who work the plantation supplied with plenty of eggs and young fryers as well as hens that have stopped laying for the stew pot.

I often wonder why Willow's great, great, great grandmother's husband, chose to call Plantation House a plantation, seeing as to how it is not in the south. I believe it would be more aptly called a farm or a ranch.    However, plantation does sound more romantic in my opinion.

Brother Thomas takes care of all the animal's health wise.    He says he had always known he wanted to be a veterinarian and that he always wants to live on the plantation.

The closer it gets to June eleventh, the more jittery the help gets. It's a great responsibility to feed and entertain so many people from Friday through Sunday, especially not knowing exactly how many are coming.

Jonathan and Thomas have transformed the grounds into a playground where everyone that wishes can play a variety of outdoor games.  Horseshoes are a favorite of the men I am told and everyone, children and all like riding the horses and playing croquet.  Some may go to the lake to swim if it is warm enough and to fish if it is not.  I know children are not as well behaved, as we were when I was a child.  They are whiney and misbehave at meals.  Parents are sparing the rod and spoiling the child as I see it.  Father would have taken us to the woodshed had any of us misbehaved, especially when others were about.

Delicious aromas are coming from the kitchen as dozens of cakes, pies and cookies are being baked for tomorrow. Hens, turkeys, hams and frying chickens are being prepared for the ovens tomorrow morning when they will cook slowly for hours. I can smell the sage and the apples with cinnamon. What a wonderful smell!

Mother's brother my Uncle Herman's brood, have started arriving. He fathered nine children and each of them had several children, now those children have children. All in all, it's getting to be a madhouse already.

Aunt Janey's children and their children begin to show up on Saturday morning. I understand there are over twenty young people connected to Aunt Janey.

Aunt Margaret's offspring and their children's children didn't arrive until Sunday morning and their group seems much better behaved. The younger ones show respect for their parents as well as for all the other adults. (A welcome change.)

I can see happy, smiling faces wherever I look. There are squealing children, harried mothers, adult males that are swearing at the horseshoes when they do not make a ringer or even get close enough to count a point. I see one of the older men talking to a couple of the players. I can't hear what is being said, but it appears as if it is some kind of an argument. I hope it isn't serious.

By mid-afternoon many of the visitors have left, leaving piles of trash lying about.

One of the smaller children fell and broke his leg. The Plantation House nurse splinted the leg and bandaged it tightly.

Only about half of the relatives came this year, but the numbers were about the same as in the past years due to so many small children. Almost every family has many grandchildren.

I'm glad we are not planning a yearly gathering or even a bi-yearly one. Perhaps a reunion every three or four years will be sufficient for everyone. Some of the relatives live in different states and it takes long tiring days to get here then to go back home.

Two of our cowhands and two of our household servants are getting married July fourth and will be gone for one week. It is not a good time for the plantation as harvest time is at hand. I guess love has no understanding of dates and work schedules.

The more I see of harried mothers and misbehaved children, the less interested I am in romance or marriage. I think I'll be like Willow. If I should get biological urges or need a friend to hold my hand, I shall seek one out.

I am now privy to all the knowledge of all the safes. It is a great responsibility and sometimes a bit scary knowing where everything is and how much cash is always in the house. The keeping of the books, having to keep each floor's expenses are kept in separate sets of ledgers. The outside expenses, materials, labor, animals vet supplies and so on, are recorded on still a separate set of books. The school is a separate deal altogether since it is a business unto itself.

Plantation House has stood in magnificent splendor since 1779, when Willow's great, great, great grandmother came into ownership of it. It had been passed down through the generations until her mother Bess, willed it to Willow.

Francious Dupea is said to have watched each board and nail applied to the construction of Plantation House ordering the builders to weed out all imperfect materials or workmanship. Only the very best was acceptable to him. The beautiful paintings on walls and ceilings were done by the finest of artists. The very best marble and wood was used in the interior of the house. He was very aware of the least infraction of workmanship and materials. Oriental carpets and soft beaver rugs covered every room with the exception of the kitchen and laundry area. Paintings of great value hang on the walls and stained glass on many of the windows. Five three story columns stand as beautiful and solid as the day they were erected. Every board, nail paint chip, putty etc. are repaired immediately upon the discovery of their imperfection inside and outside. The house is as perfect today as the day it was built. The driveway that winds through beautiful trees and flowers of made of cobblestone, causing the ride to the house to be slightly bumpy as one marvels at the breathtaking view. Huge sphinx like forms, seem to be guarding the plantation. They are situated on either side of the ornate, iron gate that separates the sculptured grounds from the plantation acreage. Fine flowerbeds and privet hedges are always in pristine condition. The other buildings including the large bunkhouse, which is by no means what other bunkhouses are like, are also kept in mint condition. The bunkhouse has a kitchen and a separate bedroom for the cook/housekeeper man that feeds all the outside help. It cannot be seen from the first floor, however one can see everything from the second and third floors of the house.

When Francious Dupea first built Plantation House, there were only five hundred acres included in the property. He however did not utilize the acreage. Evidently he had plenty of money and did not wish to mess with animals other than riding horses and milk cows, which were used to produce the milk, butter and cheese for the household.

It was Master John that had bought all the land he could convince people to part with until now. The last acreage count stood at over twenty five thousand acres after Willow's purchase of five hundred acres soon after Master John's demise. She intends to add as much acreage as she can entice property owners that border the plantation to sell. I love riding or being driven in one of the buggies to view the entire plantation and I do it as often as I can find time to do so.

We are in the process of upgrading the kitchen, putting in new, modern cookstoves, dish tubs and rebuilding cupboards. The laundry room will be next with more and larger tubs and scrub boards. A new stove for heating water will be installed as well.

Most of the tapestry covered furniture is being recovered by lighter, brighter coverings. The library chairs are to be covered with oxblood Corinthian leather. Every wall and ceiling is being cleaned and refurbished, if necessary. Willow has ordered the heavy dark drapes replaced by light pastel drapes made to order of the finest materials. Even the paintings are to be cleaned and repaired if needed.

"We are coming into a different era," said Willow "and we need to keep pace with the rest of the country."

A few days later, Willow had a heart attack. She lived only for a week before passing away.

\*\*\*\*\*\*\*\*\*\*

# CHAPTER 10

I have taken Hilda into my confidence concerning the safes and how the books are kept for each floor and the outside expenses. There has to be more than one who has knowledge in the event one of them should die. Of course both Jonathan and Thomas are aware there are safes, but do not know where they are located. The books of all the plantation business are opened for them to check at any time.

Just about a month before Willow's death, she told me about the secret passages underneath Plantation House. These were first used for wine storage then as a safe house for runaway slaves. There are also many antique pieces of furniture and solid silver serving pieces along with Ming vases and dishes from that era. There were huge tapestries rolled and wrapped in heavy cloth. I also encountered books, or journals hand printed by someone who may have been imprisoned there for a long period of time. a bed and a chamber pot still stand in the corner of a partitioned alcove. A chain is still attached to the wall through a large bolt eye. I would love to know the history of the area and perhaps will find answers in the hand printed books.

Willow's mother Bess had allowed Willow to play in these passages where she hid when her father struck her mother.

There are three entrances to the passageway. One in what are now my new quarters, one just off the hallway next to the library and one through the basement. This one is located behind what appears to be a rock wall and can be opened only by standing on something at least two feet high so that two stones in the top row can be pushed at once, exposing the entrance. Tomorrow I intend to visit the passage to investigate the books. I can hardly wait to get started.

Taking candles and a lantern with sandwiches and water to drink, I settle down to peruse the contents of the book marked, number one.

It begins, "My grandson, Francious Dupea, has imprisoned me in this dungeon and has robbed me of my worldly goods through deceit and physical torment.

Everyone believes him to be a fine man of honor. He is very believable and handsome he also is a vicious predator. I've been down here for three years now. Most of the time he brings me food and water. I have a goodly supply of food and water stored for the times he cannot or does not bring me anything. The supplies are stored in the shelves that line the wall where my chain hooks through the bolt eye. My worst problem is the sanitation, or lack thereof if Francious doesn't get here often enough. I beg him to let me go and swear I will never tell or try to regain my fortune from him, but he knows better. I would in fact, go directly to the authorities. I know I will never leave this terrible place alive. I can only pray that Francious will have to pay for his deeds very soon.

I know he has married and has a child. I hope his wife hates him and is untrue to him and that his children will hate him as well. I have repeatedly asked him for clothing but he never brings anything. My clothing is literally rotting off my body. It is fortunate for me that it never gets very cold down here. The temperature probably stays around sixty five degrees year round and I have become accustomed to that.

I fell and broke my left arm. I asked for splinting material but Francious never brought anything to even bind a board to my arm. I can only hope it heals straight. I have fashioned a sling from a pillow cover, trying to immobilize it and fuse it into place.

It is becoming longer and longer between visits from him. I feel sure he will eventually let me die from starvation. I am ill. I think I have the flu."

I picked up book number two. Wondering what time it is, I decide to take the book into my quarters to read. When I re-enter my quarters from the passage it is quiet dark outside. I look at the clock. It shows the time as nine p.m. I had been down there for seven hours, totally immersed in the sad story of the man who should have been Master of the whole plantation and everything connected with it.

Everyone has been looking for me I'm told. It was nothing too important though, just some of the help wanting to change shifts this weekend. Hilda made the decision and allowed the change just as I would have done.

I had to make some decisions on some drapery material to finish up the windows on the top floor and made a selection of materials to cover some of the heavy lounge chairs.

Jonathan informs me that we need to hire another man to help through the harvest and later to paint all of the buildings used to house the animals as well as the bunkhouse. Also the stove in the bunkhouse needs to be replaced and bed coverings are threadbare.

I am so anxious to get back to the book. However it is almost midnight before I can call it a day and I am just too tired to read any more. My head hardly hits the pillow before I am asleep. I had horrid dreams of my being chained and hung by my arms on the wall of the dungeon.

By morning light I am exhausted from the nightmares and cannot concentrate on anything. My head aches and my stomach is queasy. I've turned everything over to Hilda so I can remain in bed all day_ I cannot read because my head is pounding. I'm concerned that the prisoner, whatever his name was, may have relatives that could lay claim to Plantation House and the first five hundred acres that Francious purchased with monies that belonged to his grandfather. "Oh dear!"

I slept all day and all night and feel much better. If I dreamed, I don't remember a thing about it.

It has been a week since I was in the passage and read book number one. Harvest time is always very busy for everyone on the plantation. Maybe I can read book number two tomorrow, which is Sunday but still a workday during harvest.

I sit here with book two, hesitating to open it up afraid of what I may discover, but here goes.

"It has been nearly three weeks since Francious was here," I read. "My arm is improving but I'm running out of food and water and the sanitation is a smelly mess. Why doesn't he just kill me instead of torturing me? How can a blood relation be so cruel? I can sometimes hear voices but I can't tell where they are coming from. Perhaps I could beat on the ceiling if I could get up to it. There are some chairs down here, but I do not think I can put one on top of another in order to reach the ceiling. I might be able to tear off a board from the shelving where food was once stored, for me to pound with. I guess I may as well try, as I have nothing to lose. I am going to be dead in a few days anyway if he does not bring me food and water. I will die from the terrible stench if nothing else kills me."

"That poor man." I thought of how terrible his situation must have been and of his acceptance of his probable fate. I put the book down and went downstairs to eat dinner. Nothing seemed to have any taste. I believe I am suffering from empathy for the author of these handwritten books to the point of taste or lack or lack thereof. I seem able to feel his suffering and pain. I am so glad I am not related to Francious Dupea. He was a terrible monster.

Later I read, "I have climbed onto the chairs and I have pounded on the ceiling as hard as I can. If anyone hears me, they are not coming down here to investigate. Maybe no one except Francious knows about this place or where the entrance is located. Probably no one is even aware there is an under passage here. I'm going to try and move the chairs to a different area tomorrow, or today. I cannot tell when it is dark or daylight. I do have plenty of candles and flint. Actually boxes of them are stored down here with crates of paper to write on or to use as a taper to light candles with. All of my food is practically gone and I have water enough to last only another couple of days. I have managed to work the bolt free of the wall. However I cannot get the chain through the opening of the bolt as it is fastened around my ankle at one end and has a cross bolted to the other end. I am now able to carry the chamber pot farther down into the passageway where I empty it into a large hole and push dirt in on it. For as long as I am able I will return to this hole to relieve myself so I cannot smell the sewage as strongly."

I put the book away for the night and try to sleep. My brain just will not shut down so that I may sleep. I keep seeing him drag that chain as he makes his way to and from the sewage hole. I try to imagine how far it is to the hole and how ragged he must be and how dirty.

Why didn't his grandson come and set him free or at least give him food and water and clean clothes along with water and soap to bathe with. "Oh the monster, the horrible monster! Surely God is punishing him for his terrible crimes and his actions against his grandfather."

It is vacation time for some of the cowhands before the roundup starts. They have finished the harvest and have nearly finished with painting the buildings. They are bright and new looking and the new bedding and the cook stove is a thing of beauty.

Plantation House is looking beautiful. It is much brighter and inviting to the eye with the beautiful new drapes and upholstery. Years of smoke and dust have been cleaned from every inch of the house. Everything in the kitchen is new. We have the newest stoves made with new churns and mixing bowls and kettles that takes two persons to carry when three quarters full. The biscuit and loaf pans and huge frying pans are also new. Also new are the dishwashing tubs that will drain into large buckets to be carried outside to empty then returned to their spaces under the dish tubs. New larger work areas were installed under the cupboards and made even with the tops of the dish tubs. The laundry has been equipped with flat cloth covered boards to iron clothes on with six new irons added to the six we already have. The new stove to heat the irons on is also of the very best quality.

Jonathan and Thomas are working hard to get everything prepared for the roundup. They have purchased special clothing, boots and gloves for the men along with heavy socks, caps with earflaps and heavy flannel underpants with long legs that fit close to the body. When all the men get back from their week's vacation, they will start the roundup. It takes a long hard week to drive the animals to the stockyards. A chuck wagon will accompany the men and the men will sleep in shifts in two covered wagons. Tom, Jonathan and the cook will sleep in the chuck wagon. It's crowded but the shared body heat makes up for the discomfort. The weather is mild for this time of year. I hope it holds.

Jonathan's wife had her second baby a week ago and Thomas finally has a new baby boy.

While Jonathan, Thomas and the hands are away on roundup, I may be able to finish book two of the prisoner held for so long and under such terrible conditions. After I finish the books and find out the end result I will know if I should instigate an investigation of the allegations of the prisoner. When I think of what could happen if relatives of this man are still living and if they should bring action to reclaim this property, what will happen to all of us here at Plantation House?

Even mother was not aware of the secret passageways under the house. I believe Willow probably knew some, if not all of the history of the prisoner in the dungeon. Only when she knew she might die did she divulge the information of the secret passage. I'm hoping, praying that is not the case. I'd hate to believe either Bess or Willow would lay claim to anything that did not belong to them, especially a fortune of such magnitude. It will devastate me, all my family, as well as our people who work here on the plantation. I could just ignore what I have found, but I won't.

As I sit here in my favorite chair with book in hand, I wonder if this will be the last time I will feel like part of Plantation House. This house seems to almost be a living thing with feelings and it needs the loving care we give it.

I read, "Today I ventured into a different passageway. I can hear noises from over my head, but it is much too high here to pound on the ceiling. It's all just dirt down here, no sign of anyone ever being in this part of the passages. I will try to find another passage tomorrow. I will take along extra candles to light my way."

The writing in the book is becoming more and more shaky. The words are getting harder to read. I can visualize a filthy, ragged, skeletal man dragging a heavy chain attached to his scrawny ankle.

He was desperately trying to find a way to stay alive and to find some way out as he prayed for God to help him.

Back to the book, I continue to read. "Today I found a stairway that led to a wall made of wood. I banged on that wall for what seemed like an hour. My hands are badly bruised and bleeding. My head hurts so badly I can hardly see to write. I now know that I will never get out of here and that very soon I shall be dead. I lay down to prepare myself for death when miracle of miracles, Francious showed up. I'm sure he thought I must be dead by now. As he stared at me I saw a flicker of what I thought was shame in his eyes, but he turned and rushed away. I cried in weakness and lost hope. I just lay down to await the inevitable. I could barely hear someone coming with labored breath and I smelled food and water. I felt hands lifting my head and spooning liquid into my mouth. Water, oh how wonderful the taste. I wanted more but I was being told that I would have to go slowly or I would not be able to keep it down. I was too weak to open my eyes as I felt a warm cloth washing my face and whispered words of hope. I could smell perfume and the hands that bathed me were soft and small. I knew it was not Francious but a woman that cradled my head, washed and fed me. I could tell I was no longer in the dungeon. I was in fact in a soft bed with sweet smelling sheets. The chain was no longer around my ankle and I was clean, with a clean nightshirt covering my body. I thought I must be in heaven or that I was dreaming. A beautiful lady sat by my bed speaking quietly to me. She told me that I was all right and not to worry. She said I was safe and would remain safe. I slept."

I put the book down, unable to read further. I felt such relief that the prisoner was in safe hands at last. I put out the light and had my first good sleep in months.

The morning brought good news from the boys who had returned while I slept. The roundup had gone smoothly and we had received top dollar for our animals. They lost only two head of grown stock and half dozen head of calves that were just too small or weak to keep up. Some may survive or someone along the trail may find them and take them as their own, as is the custom.

Jonathan's wife Harriet, is all aflutter to have him home. It had only been a few days but that was much too long to be separated from him, she blushed.

Tom's wife is a little more subdued than Harriet. She isn't crazy about country ways or the quiet life compared to living in or near town. She doesn't like country style clothing and eating with students or household help. Tom is crazy about her and does not notice her shortcomings. Nor does he notice that she appears to be bored to death at family meetings or gatherings. "Two children are all I'm having," she swore. "I am not a brood sow."

Tonight I will finish book two. Hopefully I will be able to decide what to do, if anything, to find any surviving relatives of the Dupea's. I read, "Francious's wife had followed him through the passageway not knowing where he was disappearing to. She had been complaining to Francious about thumps and bumps from under the floor on several different occasions. He told her he would investigate, that maybe large rats or some other animal had somehow gotten into the walls. It was by accident that as she came into the hallway she saw him disappear into the wall. Hurriedly she caught the door before it had completely closed and had quietly followed my grandson as he made his way to where I lay almost in death.

Upon seeing me still alive he fled back the direction he had come from only to meet his wife as she stared at him. He tried to head her back to the secret panel but she would not budge. She could smell feces and hear the rattle of the chain. "What is it?" she demanded. "What is that foul stench and what is that rattling?"

"Nothing important my love. I'll attend to it later," he replied. She darted around him almost tripping over the chain that still held me. I could almost get it off over my emaciated foot, almost!

I heard her scream, "My God! What is the meaning of this? Who is this?" she demanded while trying to lift my head while screaming at her husband to, "Take that chain off his ankle and carry him upstairs."

"My health is now much improved under the care of Laura, my grandson's wife. After I had improved enough, I recounted to Laura what had happened. I found I had been in that dungeon for seven years. I hadn't any idea of what day it was or even what year since it was always dark down there. Sometimes it seems as though my imprisonment had lasted a hundred years, then at other times it is as if it only lasted months. None of that matters now. Laura has nursed me back to life and good health. I have neither seen nor spoken to Francious. Laura says he lives on the third floor with a maid and a cook, never coming downstairs for anything. I do not know what to do concerning Francious. I have only one maiden aunt. Francious and I are the last of our line so have no one to inherit. Auntie is sixty nine years of age so will never produce an heir. That leaves only Laura, who is the sweetest, most lovely woman I have ever known. Therefore, I have decided to do nothing as long as Francious stays on the third floor as my prisoner, my well cared for prisoner. I will leave everything as it now is. Laura will inherit Plantation House and all of the fortune belonging to me or to Francious at our death. I really hope he goes first. There is a chance, as I understand his health is very poor. I hate to think he would come down after my death and once again be Master of the plantation."

"Three years and seven months have passed since I was freed and my prayers have been answered. Francious died last night as we slept, I know not of what malady. Now I can die in peace. I am seventy nine years old. My health is about normal for a man of my age. I'm tired and I'm ready to meet my maker." It was signed, "Pierre Dupea."

What a load off my mind. Plantation House and we are safe.

**********

# CHAPTER 11

Jonathan stands by Thomas, resting his wide shoulders against the corral. Looking at Thomas's gray hair makes him realize how old Tom is, how old they both are.

"It's been a great life," John said.

"Yes it has. I've always been happy here. I can think of no other place I'd rather be," Tom agrees.

Some ten years back, Jonathan had asked Thomas, "How are your boys leaning toward making their lives here, or do any of them want to go someplace else?"

Tim replied, "Well, I'm not quite sure about Henry but Cecil is like me. He loves the cattle and the land. Mary Ellen will probably get married and leave I suppose."

That is how it has played out. The eldest sons of Jonathan and Thomas followed in their father's footsteps. The rest of the children have decided to travel and see what the rest of the world is like before they decide where or what they want to do for the rest of their lives.

Jonathan and Thomas thought this was a good idea. They all needed to visit many places and meet a lot of people. It wasn't anything either of them would want to do, "The young folks are very different these days. All we ever wanted to do was to get through school as quickly as possible and get started to work," Thomas laughed.

Simpson had passed away two years past after a short illness. Everyone mourned him very much. He was like family and he had loved every inch of the plantation. Simpson had started out as gardener when he was just a teenager. Miz Bess had hired him in spite of Master John saying, "No!" He had worked as a gardener until he was put to work in the sowing of the wheat and hay grasses. He later fit right in with the cattle roundups. Timmy had become groundskeeper after he and Minnie had married.

Plantation House now employs eight full time men that take care of everything that needs caring for.

*********

# CHAPTER 12

It is storm time again, time for tornados, floods and later snow and ice. Plantation House is never troubled by floods and seldom with strong winds. However severe snow and ice storms become we can now deal with them better. We now haul with four wheel jeeps instead of wagons. There are now several hay and grain enclosures over the plantation so the men have only to drive to each station to get feed to the animals. They cannot do anything about the freezing weather but have learned to keep all of the animals in the most southern part of the grazing lands in storm season. There has never been another ice storm like the one in the grandfather's time. Plantation House stands strong and inviting with little or no evidence of deterioration with any and all repairs kept done.

Jonathan's eldest son Michael took over when Jonathan retired as Thomas's son Cecil filled his own father's niche. Both boys are doing wonderful jobs.

When Mike retired, at a somewhat earlier age than his father had, his second son Patrick fit right into the managerial spot. When Cecil retired as vet, his son Jack took over in his place.

Everything is mechanized now. We have new tractors, jeeps, electric power, indoor plumbing and most of the cash is in the bank now with CD's and long-term bonds.

Nearly all drive his or her own automobile and some can fly the twenty four seat plane that was purchased by Mike, Jonathan's son, to be used for everything needed at Plantation House.

"Patrick, has anyone decided the exact date to hold the family reunion?" inquired Jack.

"Yes, it is to be June tenth, just after school dismisses for the summer. Hey Patrick do you remember that reunion when we were ten or eleven when Grandfather came down on both our dad's for cursing the game when they were playing horseshoes?"

"Yep, I sure do. Dad swore at the horseshoes saying, Get around that peg you son of a bitch and your dad called them bastards when his throw would go wild. Man did the two of them ever get it." Patrick was laughing so hard he started to hic-cup.

"What would Grandpa think if he could hear today's language in just normal conversation?" asked Jack.

"Well, I guess we had better get the men busy for the roundup and we need to get the information out to the buyers so they can make their bids on the cattle. Now that's a lot different. The old way we had to drive the herd to the stockyards. Now the buyers haul the cattle to market in huge semi trucks. Much better this way," they agreed.

Thousands of head of cattle were driven to the north pastures nearest the barns. We feed them to keep them from wanting to head back to the south pastures where they spend most of their time.

The cowhands were whistling and singing to move the cattle along. They were twirling their ropes and saying, "Get your ass back there you stupid mother fucker." Someone else yelled out, "Morey, get those sons a bitches back in the herd before they get ahead of us."

The bulls were kept separate from the rest of the herd. Plantation House sold only the culls, those that were too old or too runty or had gotten injured somehow. Calves that were old enough to be weaned were corralled in fenced enclosures to be culled. Some were animals to keep for a good bloodline and the others were to be sold.

The younger calves were kept with their mothers until the last minute when they would be sold separately to restaurants and hotels to be served as veal. They had never eaten anything except milk from their mother's teets. All of the animals were in good condition from what Jack and Pat saw. This should be a great year.

Saturday brought many bidders who brought trucks along to haul their expected purchases. The buyers knew these cattle had not been held without water until the last moment. They were then allowed to drink their fill, as some and maybe most of the sellers did when they sold by the pound on the hoof.

Plantation House has the best reputation anywhere. Everything we sell is guaranteed to be as advertised. Whether it be beef, horses, swine or produce, only the very best is good enough to bear the Plantation House logo.

All week buyers were coming and going, hauling truckloads of beef. Some three thousand animals were already gone. Ton's of alfalfa and clover hay are being bought by those who have herds they must feed during the winter.

The last load of hogs had been carted off along with the veal calves and a party was getting underway. There would be no hard liquor, just beer and lots of food and music by a great local band for dancing.

Wives of the cowhands along with kitchen help joined the merrymakers. The students could stay out until just before dark at which time they had to return to their quarters. Plantation House always strove to protect the reputations of the students. Now, in this new generation, the girls complain. Younger and younger girls were experienced even before enrolling in Grover School for Girls. However the teachers and housemothers still insist upon following the rules. They feel as though they must protect their girls as the school has for generations.

Some of the students could be overheard grumbling and swearing, (very unladylike) that, "This damned school is stuck in the dark ages. Doesn't anyone here know this is the twentieth century? Shit! We'll be old fuckers before we even get laid."

One of the girls was overheard saying, "These damned uniforms are for the birds too. Everyone dressing alike went out of style many years ago. I'm not coming back here next year I don't care what Father says."

A tall seventeen year old yelled, "What could they do to us if we just went back to the party, kill us?"

"Oh I don't think anything quite so drastic as that is going to happen," said Miz Volt, the teacher. "However the party is winding down. The fellows have to be back on the job by seven a.m. Now lets get ready for bed. Tomorrow is another school day. Groans and nasty remarks followed Miz. Volt as she closed the door smiling, "Oh, to be young again," she whispered.

The next morning everything seemed to be back to normal except for one cowhand. He quit to, as he put it, "Spend my money on wine, women, song and partying."

"Changes, changes!" Jack observed. "Years past when one was employed by Plantation House, they stayed for life. Now help comes and goes."

"Yeah, it's a new way O.K. and I can't blame them too much. There is a lotta world out there to see and a lotta money to be made," Patrick mused.

"Do you ever get the urge to join the flow and do something else?" Jack inquired.

"Nope, not me. I like what I do and I like the life. I'd never want to be anywhere other than here."

"By the time our children are old enough, do you think any of them will want to stay here and run the place? I mean, as it has been run in the past_ by family?"

"Well, I guess we better have large families so some of them will be bound to want to stay," Patrick laughed.

"My wife says she's having only two and that's it. How does Viola feel about kids?"

"Well," Patrick replied, "Vi hasn't said up to now. However we already have three so it's up to you to catch up," slapping Jack on the back.

Patrick had married Viola Small just after graduation. His first son was born just ten months later. He was lucky because Vi loved the plantation and the life it afforded.

Martha, Jack's wife, wasn't nearly as fond of country living as Vi was and she had no intention of having kids one after the other. She wanted to travel and take in all the wonders of the world. Being stuck with a house full of children did not appeal to her in the least.

**********

# CHAPTER 13

This past December and this January are reminiscent of the ice storm in Tom and Nellie's time but much easier to cope with. Jeeps go anywhere in all kinds of weather and feeding was a much easier fete having the storage of hay and grain to feed from. Nonetheless some three hundred animals perished in the cold. Again, many of the beefs were skinned out and the meat salvaged for house meat and tons were distributed to food banks and to any individuals that came and helped with the skinning and butchering. The beef had all been frozen and only the upper legs, haunches and the flesh down the back were harvested. As soon as it thawed, the carcasses were bulldozed into huge trenches cut by the backhoes.

Everyone worked long hard days for three weeks. It was a cold backbreaking job with fingers so cold the men could not make them work. Jack had bought each of them hand warmers and twenty below socks and lace up boots, but their fingers were still too cold to work well.

The kitchen help were worn out as well. They prepared huge pots of steaming rich soups for thermos bottles and gallons of hot coffee, making many extra dishes, pots and pans to wash. The men all ate in the kitchen at the long table used for household help. Usually the outdoor help ate at the bunkhouse kitchen. They had access to the same foods as the indoor employees, but prepared by a Chinese male cook that had been with Plantation House for many years. Chen came to the kitchen to help prepare food and drink, for 'his family' and to load up the food to be taken into the field. Some men had stayed to watch over the cattle while others came in to eat and warm up then they would trade places so all could take turns for nourishment and to get warm all the way through.

Electric wires were frozen and broke under the weight of the ice. It left the house with no lights and no power to run the electric coffee pots, deep fat fryers and so on. Patrick had prepared for this by having a huge generator installed some years past and had recently hired an electrician to stay on the plantation through the storm time.

Before the thaw set in tempers were frazzled and several of the help came down with the flu. There was lots of coughing, runny noses, earaches, sore throats, chills and fevers putting that much more pressure on those that were well.

Some of the students had runny noses and coughs as well. A couple of them had not returned from Christmas vacation. They had decided to finish their educations in local colleges. Hormones raging and the strict rules of Grover School for Girls at Plantation House were just to hard for some of today's youth to accept.

Jack and Patrick were worn down to a crawl. They spent many more grueling hours laboring than any of the rest of the help did, having to be everywhere at the same time.

"Man, if we get through this storm without going crazy I'm taking a couple of weeks off and go to some warm island and get reacquainted with my wife," Jack swore.

"Sounds like a winner to me. Maybe Vi and I can go when you get back."

Just dreaming of those warm beaches gave Jack more strength to get through each day.

Patrick heard someone saying, "Shit! Shit! Shit!" in a painful voice. Hurrying to the man he saw blood streaming from a deep gash on the man's right hand.

"What happened Dave?" asked Pat as he took a clean handkerchief from his pocket and tied it around the wrist to serve as a tourniquet while pressing a second one to the wound. "Come on Dave. I'll get ya to the house where you can be taken care of. It's gonna be O.K. Loosen up that tourniquet once in a while, while I drive."

In the birthing room at the house Dave was being tended by Roxanne, the best nurse around. She was a twenty six year old single lady from Bakersfield California. Dave seemed not to notice his injury as much as he did Roxanne.

"There now! You are going to be just fine. I've put in four stitches to hold the wound together. It will heal with hardly a scar," she told Dave.

"How about a movie after this ice is gone?" suggested Dave.

"Umm, we will see. You just take care of that hand for right now," she told him.

Dave felt fine leaving the house. Roxanne hadn't said no and he was pretty sure she would say yes soon. Life on the plantation could get weary for young folks if they didn't have friends of the opposite sex and if one enjoyed country life, it could be hard to find a mate.

\*\*\*\*\*\*\*\*\*

# CHAPTER 14

All the students had gone home for the summer except for three. They were Wanda Sprigg, Nancy Olson and Tammy Long, whose parents almost never visited them or had them home for the holidays. Plantation House has always accepted the unhappy girls, giving them special attention to make up for what they felt as rejection.

Everyone on the plantation had worked their buns off to get everything ready for the family reunion. Jack and Patrick were looking forward to seeing their siblings and hearing all about their travels.

On Friday night family started arriving. Some were very tired and some were very lively. Laughter could be heard all over the place. Wonderful aromas from the kitchen made mouths water in anticipation. The ballroom had been set up to feed the group and bands could be heard playing soft music from surround sound speakers.

The students empty bedrooms were being used to sleep many along with the first and second floor bedrooms being opened up.

Extra Kitchen help was hired to keep the food flowing. If it didn't rain Sunday there would be a huge Bar-B-Q to feed everyone outside.

Six horseshoe game areas were pegged and waiting. A baseball diamond and a croquet space were set up. There were riding horses ready for whomsoever may care to ride. Indoors, in Willow's old quarters, table games were waiting along with instruments to be played for those so inclined.

Dancing and live music took up half the ballroom. If one didn't see something they liked, just asked. If it could be found, it would be provided.

"Well did ya have a great experience and where all did ya travel?" Patrick demanded to hear from the brothers and cousins that followed him and Jack around the barn looking over the animals.

Jasper spoke up saying, "Brother Pat it was great and I'm going back, or at least going to a different country soon. I think I liked Dublin the best. I like the people, the food and the ale. They have the happiest music found anywhere. We went to the Kissing Rock, or the Blarney Stone if you prefer. People were happily being lifted, or held I guess it would be, to kiss the stone. They raise beautiful horses and we went to a factory where they made fine lace. Of course Ginger had to buy yards of it. We went through the brewery which I must say was smelly but the brew was great and it doesn't take much of it to knock ya on yer ass."

Jeffery said, "The wife and I really liked London except for the food. All the great cathedrals and the wax museum and the changing of the guard are spectacular. We enjoyed the live theater and the nightspots with skits performed by loud actors in brightly colored costumes. They still have places where the Can-Can is performed. That was great also."

"How about you Samson?" Jack asked. "Are ya going back or will ya go someplace else?"

"Naw. I think I've had enough traveling to last me for sometime. I also perfer women from the U.S.A. Somehow I just didn't cotton to anyone I met. I liked seeing the animals and seeing how people do things in France as opposed to how we do it here. I liked watching the floor shows and tried many of the foods that everyone told me was the best food in the world. No way! It is so rich for the most part and very expensive. Give me a drumstick off a young rooster every time.

The art galleries were wonderful and so were their cathedrals and churches, but I guess I feel closer to God in a small church right here."

Raymond chimed in saying, "I guess I feel like Samson does. It's nice to have gone once so you can say you've been there and it was educational. Anyway I was taught there is no place like home. I won't be traveling for quite some time, if ever. Oh maybe here in the good ol' U.S.A. where there are hundreds of interesting things to see here and in every other state."

I think the wives are more interested in traveling than we fellers are only not such long stays. Maybe a month out of each year would satisfy them and traveling with children is a drag. They get bored or have a belly ache or need to go to the bathroom when there is none around," opined Jeffery.

In the house the women were chattering a mile a minute oooing and ahhing at the clothes and jewelry the women had brought back.

"Oh kid, you should see the dress shops. They handle beautiful merchandise and EXPENSIVE! Man they are that. Too much for more than one outfit, at least for me," Vivian, Jeffery's wife said.

"Any of you gonna live on the plantation and work in the running of the place?" asked Pat.

"I'm ready to settle down and take my responsibility here," Samson stated, "and it can't be too soon for me."

"Me too," Raymond agreed. "There just ain't no place I'd rather be and no work I'd like better than this."

Patrick and Jack smiled at each other.

The plantation was a happy place again until a fight broke out over a horse. One cousin had saddled a horse and another cousin rode off on the animal. The young boys were pretty well matched so the men just let them bang around on each other for a while before breaking them up when the women began to scream for someone to do something. Both boys had bloody noses and each looked as though an eye may turn black.

By three p.m. many of the people were heading home. For the most part everyone looked happy, wearing smiles saying what a good time they had, had. The two boys that had fought were smiling and slapping each other on the back, friends again.

Employees were glad for the reprieve from long hours of labor. They were happy because they knew they would be receiving a hefty bonus in their paychecks. Monday was cleanup time indoors as well as outside. It always amazed the help that the guests just dropped garbage or left plates where ever they finished with them. There were trash containers every few feet outside and a number of waste baskets throughout every room that most never used.

\*\*\*\*\*\*\*\*\*

# CHAPTER 15

I Patrick, finally opened and read aunt Gracie's letters that she had instructed not to be opened unless we had not heard from her for seven years. After reading them I investigated the secret passages underneath Plantation House.

Father had turned everything over to me and Jack years back after aunt Gracie had been declared legally dead instructing us not to open them until after his death. If Father had ever examined the passageways or read the journals, he never mentioned it to anyone. When he passed on he had left strict instructions as to how those particular papers and letters were to be handled saying, "Keep the secrets of Plantation House even from your wives and children until it is time for you to choose the one person you have unlimited faith in. It must be one that will best care for and keep Plantation House secrets that are better kept from others in the family as well as the general public."

I have done as my father instructed. Now I must choose the next keeper of Plantation House and her secrets. The following is what I found in aunt Gracie's journals from all those years past when I was just a small boy and Plantation House was very different. Now when Samson and Timmy take over one of them will be keeper of all things, Plantation House and her secrets which follow.

\*\*\*\*\*\*\*\*\*\*

# CHAPTER 16

Aunt Gracie wrote this; "I am just back from the attorney that handles Plantation House legal business. It was the new partner in the firm of Windsor, Green, Kerney and Smith, Smith being the new man on the block, that helped me today. Fredric Smith was tall, black hair, one dimple in his left cheek and blue eyes that seemed to be holding a secret that was eager to be let out. His wide smile intrigued me causing little ripples of pleasure that covered my body. I smiled all the way home wondering what kind of excuse I could give to need further input from a legal angle.

Later as I move about my duties humming, I'll be down to get you in a taxi honey, Hilda's eyebrows raised and her mouth widened in a big smile. "Me thinks milady Gracie has met a gentleman she likes."

"Now how could you believe such a thing?" I scolded as one plump index finger pecked her forehead and she winked.

Days have passed, still I can think of no excuse to call or visit the office of Fredric Smith. Damn!!

The telephone in the main living room at the foot of the stairs rang loudly as I made my way to pick it up. "Gracie of Plantation House," I spoke into the mouthpiece.

"Just who I was looking for," a somewhat familiar voice said. "I was wondering if I could come by and get your signature on some papers? Oh, by the way this is Fred Smith," he added.

"Of course Mr. Smith. When would you like to come by?"

"Is this afternoon too soon?"

"Fine, come by at three p.m. if that is convenient for you."

"See you then," he said.

"I have time to bathe, rest a little then dress in something nice before he shows up," I think to myself.

My heart is racing, my palms are damp. I don't know just why I am so nervous, after all it is only a man. However I have never had any contact with a male person except in very impersonal ways, socially, business, school and so forth. Here I am, forty nine years of age and acting like a school girl over a man I've met only once and is probably fifteen years my junior.

I see the car pull up, it must be him. I have no other appointments with anyone today. I open the door slowly somehow fearing to see Fredric Smith again but sure I'd run to him if he decided to turn away. He is carrying a Gucci attache case, Italian leather shoes, his suit didn't come off any rack nor did the tie he wore. Seeing him close up I could see some gray sprinkled through his hair and tiny laugh lines around his eyes. He was not as young as I had thought.

I have tiny crustless sandwiches ready on the coffee table. Pouring the tea I asked, "What papers did I miss signing while I was at the office?"

"Oh nothing important. Actually nothing. I just needed an excuse to call on you."

"An excuse…Why?"

"I wasn't sure you would want to see me so I invented papers that needed your signature."

"Well, here we are. Would you like a guided tour around the place or would you rather sit here and get acquainted?"

"Here is fine with me if it is with you," he stated.

"All right, fill me in on who you are. Where are you from and are you married or otherwise entangled?"

"You know my name, Fredric Smith and you know where I work. I'm not married or spoken for. I just celebrated my forty sixth birthday. I was born in Brooklyn, New York, my parents are dead and I have no siblings. I like classical music and love to dance. I was married once when I was in college but it didn't last. Now it's your turn."

"You already know my history along with Plantation House, I've never been married and I've never even had a gentleman friend. I've never wanted one up till now. I like red meat, biscuits and gravy, cream pies, chocolate cake, fast cars and I love riding a good horse. I spent several years in France studying art and I'm pretty good at it. I play violin, piano, flute and the harp. I do those pretty well also. Is there anything else you would like to know?" I asked.

"Yes. I'd like to know if you will take in a movie with me or dinner or both…soon?"

"I'm free this weekend," I offered.

"O.K. that's a date.  Pick you up around six p.m. Saturday?" he asked, taking my hand in his for just a moment before he left.

This week is flying by.  I'm glad it will soon be Saturday.  I know I will never forget my first date.  I have not spoken of the event with Jonathan, Patrick or Jack.  If he never asks me for another date no one will be teasing me or feeling sorry for me.

I'm wearing my yellow linen suit with a fitted top and shoes to match.  I hope he likes me.  We went to the movies first so we could have time for a few dances at the dinner club just outside of town.  I'm glad we went there.  The food was great and the seating was scarce so we had to be seated in a small corner space where our bodies touched from time to time.  As we danced on the tiny dancefloor Fredric held me close.  I loved his cologne and his strong arms around me.  The ride home was wonderful.  Still holding hands, we talked about just everything.  Fredric was up on current events as well as being well informed on the political shenanigans of the oval office.

Still holding onto my hand Fredric walked me to my door and although I waited for a kiss, it did not come.  Instead he stepped back, released my hand and bade me goodnight. I'm wondering if I did something to turn him off, as the young folks say, or if he just didn't take a liking to me. Wellll...it is a little late in my life to think of attracting a hunk like Fredric.

It's Wednesday, Fredric hasn't called.

Friday I answered the doorbell to find a blue uniformed delivery person holding a huge bouquet of red roses. Going to the table drawer by the phone, I extracted some bills to tip the young man. Included was a card which read, "Will you accompany me tomorrow for dinner and a show? Please say yes, Fred." His phone number was on the business card that had also been included.

This time I'm wearing an off the shoulder dinner dress made of beige slipper satin, with heels and a diamond clip that matches my ear rings. I'm not a sleek young skinny thing but I'm still in pretty good shape. If he doesn't get stirred up with all this bare shoulder and cleavage...well he is a man isn't he?

Today Fredric is wearing a white evening jacket with black trousers. The front of his white shirt is ruffled. He is wearing diamond cuff links and black Italian slip on shoes. He is so handsome.

"Hey babe, you are looking good," he said.

"You look pretty spiffy yourself," I returned.

As soon as we were seated in the front seat of his Lincoln he suddenly reached over and kissed me full on the lips. Laughing he said, "Take that!" and drove very fast over our newly run cement drive or maybe it's called concrete. The cobblestone drive that was replaced was pretty but not very smooth and it had taken a lot of repair to keep it as usable as it was beautiful.

Fred, as he prefers to be called, is an active man. He wants to dance every dance and when we are at a restaurant he sits on the same side as I do so he can smooth my hair, touch my face, flick imaginary lint from my dress, etc. He will sometimes stop the car, run around to my side of the car, lift me out and pull me along to see something or just to walk for awhile. He is talkative and asks too many questions about personal things concerning Plantation House and those who run it as well as how everything is done. At first I filled him in on a few things but now I do not divulge much that is not apparent to the naked eye. Oh, did I tell you? He finally got around to kissing me thoroughly, leaving me breathless and shaking like a rabbit. When I open my eyes and look into his after a kiss, I see that same glint that seems to have some secret just bursting to get out. He breathes so hard when we kiss but I believe he may be pretending, at least somewhat.

On our fourth date, Fred suggested a motel. Even though I want to experience sex and lovemaking at least once in my life, I hesitate to go all the way. Fred just seems too sure of himself. I'm way past the time of getting pregnant so that isn't the reason. I don't know exactly what is the matter with me.

Fred has been giving me small presents, a gold cigarette lighter, a charm bracelet, a five pound box of imported chocolates and a couple of fabulous silk scarves. Maybe he thinks he can sweet talk me into something more than a casual relationship. If I decide to try on the sex thing it will be for me, not for anything Fred says or does.

I decided after some thought that on this Saturday's date I will agree to go to a hotel or motel for sex. I've thought and thought about it and can come up with no good reason to deny myself. No matter what Fred's motive is I hope he knows a lot about the act because I don't know a darned thing.

When Fred came to pick me up this evening I said, "Why don't we pass on the theater and dinner and go to that hotel or motel you have suggested before?"

Fred was shocked, or at least looked shocked. It didn't take any coaxing. He drove to one of the best places in town, if the advertisements don't lie.

"Would you like me to order up some champagne or a bite to eat?" he asked.

"No. I want to be aware of every moment of my first sexual experience," I said as I slipped out of my jacket. Fred looked perplexed but rallied nicely. Unbuttoning my dress in back he lifted it over my head, he then took my hands and placed them at his shirt buttons as he was reaching behind my back to unhook my bra.

My fingers tremble as I try to unfasten his buttons. Then he put my hands on his belt buckle. I can feel the heat from his body while I shake as if I'm having a chill. Finally getting the belt undone I just stand there until he put my hand on his zipper. Somehow I'm standing here nude except for my panties and sling pumps. I feel a great need to grab the sheet and wrap it around my body. Fred's trousers are in a heap on the floor leaving him in only his under shorts, socks and loafers. He is planting little kisses on my face and ears. His hands are running up and down my bare sides and stomach. Quickly he sheds his shorts and shoes and socks and slides my panties down over my hips to the floor. By now I am getting very aroused and it is very evident that Fred is as well. Fred isn't saying a word but he seems to be in the mood and becomes more excited as he touches my breast and trails kisses down my belly.

"I can't wait!" he exclaims. "I've got to have you now," and he slid his member into that secret place causing me to cry out as the hymen broke and later as thrills flowed through my entire body, not once but several times. As Fred rolled off me onto the bed he choked out, "Damn! You weren't lying. You never have had a man before. I thought you were just giving me a line as a lot of women do."

I'm not saying anything but I'm thinking a mile a minute. "So this is what all the talk is about. Not too bad but I'm thinking it would be…well different…more something. Maybe next time, if there is a next time."

"Gracie, I'm crazy about you. Why don't we get married?"

"Married?" I almost yelled. "I've never wanted to be married."

"What do you mean you don't want to get married? Don't you love me?"

"I—I don't think so. I like you well enough and I enjoy being with you but that's all."

Fred didn't call for three weeks but even if he had I couldn't have seen him. One of the cowhands has come down with some illness. We don't know what it is and it looks as though a couple of more men are coming down with the same thing. Until we find out what it is we will keep all indoor help inside and not allow the cowhands to come near the house. I remember being told about the diphtheria spreading until we lost three or more. I can't remember right off how many it was. Anyway we do not want any kind of disease spreading all over the plantation. I'm filling in first at one job then at another. I'm so tired I just drop into bed or go to sleep while still on my feet.

Now it's raining and blowing, breaking limbs off trees and tearing shingles off the barns and other buildings. The chickens have all gone to roost and it is only three p.m. The clouds are rumbling and black. It looks as though we are in for a real downpour.

Chin Chan has come down with whatever the hands have. The doctor doesn't know what they have but is prescribing antibiotics, aspirin, lots of liquids and chicken soup. He says the medicinal value comes from the chickens feet, so we scald the feet, cut off the nails and skin the outside of the leg and feet boiling them with veggies.

I was up in the hayloft throwing down hay by the pitchfork full when I slipped and sprained my ankle. Now I'm of very little use to anyone. When Fred did call, upon finding out that I am laid up and the hands are ill he came right out, saying he is going to play nurse until I can get around. I've tried to convince him to leave but he refuses. He says he has vacation time due and is taking it now while his case load is light.

I've been feeling very upset and am having a discharge. My back aches and my lower abdomen hurts a lot as well. I think I'm going to have the doctor examine me. I can't seem to shake this thing. Maybe it's whatever the hands have. They are getting well, or better at least so I guess I'll survive if I do have it.

Dr. Foley came to my quarters and examined me asking many questions that I do not quite understand. "What do you think the trouble is Doctor?"

Doctor Foley coughed into his hand looking uncomfortable before he spoke. "Gracie I must ask you this and I apologize for asking, but have you had sexual contact with anyone lately?"

"Why do you ask that Doctor?"

"Because I'm afraid you may have a venereal disease. I will take a swab sample to the laboratory for testing but I'm afraid that will only verify my diagnosis."

"Yes, I had my first and only sexual experience about four weeks ago."

"Your first ever?"

"Yes, my first."

Doctor Foley looked shocked and asked, "Who…Who was the person you had this experience with? I'll have to contact him so he can get medical attention as well. I'm going to give you a shot and leave a prescription at the drug store for you. Be sure to take them exactly as I have prescribed and take the entire prescription."

It's too bad the doctor has to inform Fred. I wish his damned thing would rot off. I'll get even with that man one way or another.

I asked the doctor not to tell Fred I had contracted the disease. I don't want him to take flight before I have a chance to find a way to make him pay for the dirty deed he has done.

As soon as I was able I went into town and bought several items I will need…soon.

My ankle is well and I am feeling my old self again. Fred called yesterday. He hesitated when he hears my voice, waiting I suppose too see if I had contracted his venereal disease. I pretended everything is great and that my ankle had mended. I invited him to dinner in my quarters and ask him to pick up a large water cooler, a five gallon one at least.

We ate sirloin steaks, green beans, salad and a large slab of chocolate cake. Everything tasted wonderful. I served wine from my personal wine closet and handed a glass of it to Fred. I poured myself one and pretended to sip at it.

"Fred, come with me. I want to let you in on a little secret of Plantation House," I smiled.

Eagerly he followed me to the bookcase at the end of the fireplace. I pushed the secret latch opening the entrance into the passageway that leads to the dungeon where Francious had held his grandfather prisoner for seven years. By now Fred is stumbling as he follows me, still drinking from his wine glass.

"Say!" he says, "This is neat. What do you keep down here?"

"Umm, this and that," I tell him as we come into sight of the bed with new sheets, pillows, cases, blankets and even a soft comforter. There is a bedside table with a few aspirin, band-aids, iodine, antibiotic cream and lots of pens, pencils and paper. A long shelf with many and varied kinds of canned foods and a can opener also has a small micro wave, an electric coffee pot, plastic tableware and paper plates and cups. I had purchased a chemical toilet and a whole case of toilet paper and even a small television. I would have bought a small refrigerator but I couldn't have gotten it down here alone and no one must know about this place, especially since dear Fred will be down here for a very long time.

The long chain fastened to a foot square by fifteen foot stud that is one of the supports for the ceiling or my bedroom subflooring. The other end of the chain I have fastened to Fred's right ankle as he sleeps peacefully from the drug I placed in his wine. When he awakens he will find he has everything needed to survive. I'm leaving a note that reads, "A man that carries around gonorrhea and gives it to a woman on her first sexual experience does not deserve to be amongst the rest of human kind. There are more electrical bulbs in the box by the lamp. I will always see to it that you have food and water. Don't bother to pound on anything to try and attract attention. It is soundproof down here. Have a nice time. Oh yes, there are many changes of clothes, pajamas, shoes, extra bedding etc. in the trunk where the candles are kept should the electric ever go off also a flashlight with extra batteries. G.

It has been five days since I placed Fred in the dungeon and I am going to check on him tonight. I've given him some time to become familiar with his new home. I hope he is very unhappy.

My basket that I carry has some goodies from the kitchen, fried chicken, a big salad, fruit mix and cream pie. If he behaves I will put them within his reach. If he does not, I will put them just out of reach to torment him.

I have never, up to now, been able to understand how Francious could have imprisoned anyone let alone his own grandfather. Now I can understand hating someone so strongly that one can take pleasure from the power you have over your enemy. Of course Francious's motivation was strictly monetary and it was after all his grandfather, I try reasoning to myself.

After locking my front entrance I walk to the passageway to where my prisoner awaits. I can hear him moving about as his chain clinks away.

"Hello dear heart," I greet him. "How are you feeling? Are you ready for some treats?"

Fred sat on the side of the bed dressed in the same clothes he was wearing when I left him five days hence. He was shaved, his hair was combed and I could see he had been reading. Speaking through tight lips glaring at me Fred demanded, "Gracie get this chain off me and let me out of here. What the hell do you think you are doing? This is kidnapping pure and simple. You will go to prison for this."

"Nope, I don't think so."

"Do you believe you are above the law?"

"Nope, but you aren't leaving here alive to tell anyone and no one except me even knows this place exists. How do you think the law is going to find out about this?"

"Gracie, my car is here. Don't you know someone is going to figure something is wrong and investigate?"

"My dear Fred, don't you think I thought of that? I took my bike and left it behind some bushes where I drove your car to, with gloves on, and left it. I then rode my bicycle home. It was three o'clock in the morning and no one saw me. However I did dress myself in black slacks and shirt with a wide brimmed hat in case anyone should have seen a figure in the dark they would believe it was a man. Now settle down and enjoy your meal. Why haven't you changed clothes. I told you there are several changes in the trunk."

"Sure! Change my trousers over this chain. Good trick if I could manage it."

I had completely forgotten about that. Now how is he going to change clothes, his pants and underwear. I wentupstairs and got some of the powder I had put into his wine. I will have to put him out before I can remove the chain to bathe and change him.

"I know you must be starving for something other than canned stuff so eat up," I ordered.

Fred shot a hate filled look at me but dug into the food with gusto. I had been able to get the drug into the tall glass of tea I knew he liked, waiting for it to take effect. I watched as he ate the last crumb of the cream pie. I can see that he is getting sleepy. He takes one last swig of the iced tea and lays over on the bed.

I transfer the chain to his wrist just to be safe. He could possibly wake up before I finish. My, his body is beautiful. I must remember to bring some bar bells down here so he can keep in shape. I'd hate to see this beautiful man turn to flab.

I have finished his sponge bath and changed his clothes. He looks and smells better now. I'm leaving before he wakes. He needs to know this is going to be his home from now on.

\*\*\*\*\*\*\*\*\*

## CHAPTER 17

Jonathan and Harriet came to visit today, mostly they keep to themselves. Like me they are graying and a little less active as the years pass. Our visit is a pleasant one. I have filled both of them in on the locations of the safes and where to find important papers should anything happen to Hilda and me.

Jonathan has always had access to the books and can now write checks on bank accounts belonging to the plantation as a whole. He does not have any knowledge of the dungeon or the history of Francious. I must make sure someone has that history along with how to enter the passageways. I guess I'll leave a sealed envelope containing my will along with everything I know about Plantation House.

Fred's car was found but no trace of him. The police are still questioning and searching. Newspapers carry the case day after day.

Jonathan has approached me and some of the others in the family regarding buying the extra thousand acres for sale to our north. The

Flints are old and have outlived their children. There is now no one left to inherit the ranch so they are selling.

The main goal of Plantation House has always been to enlarge the acreage. That being the case we all agree to make an offer on the Flint place including the house and outbuildings which can house families who work for the plantation. That would give better access and less mileage to get hands to handle the far side of the land and animals.

We won't use money from the safes. We will need proof of what we pay for the land and to keep records of all the expenditures for tax information that the government now keeps close tabs on.

Jack and his wife now have three boys even though she had said she was only going to have two children. "Sometimes slips do count," Jack laughed.

The men are preparing for a coyote hunt. We are losing too many young calves and even some mature cattle. However Patrick believes a big cat is the culprit and not the coyotes. We were required to buy a permit from the game department after showing them evidence of the cattle losses we and the neighbors have suffered.

Lightning struck one of the hay storage enclosures burning all the feed and several hundred acres of pasture land. The men set backfires to keep the flames from spreading. we are lucky, the wind did not come up. We could have lost forest land as well as buildings had the wind changed directions or velocity.

As of late it seems we have some kind of confrontation between the students or between teacher and student everyday. We finally gave in on the dress code allowing the students to choose between dresses and slacks or skirts and blouses. They must choose colors that are not overly loud and they must come from the schools supply of clothing. No short shorts or skirts above the knees will be accepted nor will plunging necklines.

We are considering closing down the school. Today's young people are just too hard to handle. Parents are asking us to please reconsider. They fear public schools and except for Catholic schools there is the same problem everywhere including foreign finishing schools for the young ladies. I'm amazed at the behavior of today's children and young adults. Many seem to have no definite understanding of where they wish to go nor of what to do if they get there.

Here on the plantation we often hire men to work only to find out they do not intend to wade in cowshit for any damn job and they leave. What their perception of working on a farm is, I do not know. I do know however that good help is hard to come by even if one pays a very good wage.

It is the same with the house staff. People will apply for work with a long list of, 'I do not do's'. Although we have automatic dishwashers, that is one of the most frequent, do nots. Laundry is the same and vacuuming is a big no-no as well. They might dust, make beds or stack canned food on shelves. We are fortunate to have Hilda and some of her relatives who are good un-complaining workers. Hilda is getting on in age but is still a great co-ordinator. She keeps the entire house humming in tune. She does the hiring and firing of household help, I'm so happy to say.

Our number three kitchen helper's boyfriend came to the kitchen and ordered Alice to leave with him. When she did not go along with him he pulled her outside and beat her with his fists and kicked her.

Hilda believing he would kill Alice banged the boyfriend over the head with a length of firewood. The fellows from the barn saw part of the action and ran over and escorted the beast off the plantation telling him not to come back or Hilda's firewood would be nothing compared to what they would do to him.

Alice had two broken ribs where the bastard had kicked her and one of her front teeth was just hanging. I quickly pushed the tooth back into place and dosed it with a pain killer to lessen the pain as I loaded her into my car and rushed her to the hospital. While the doctors were tending her I went to the police station and registered a complaint against Jeb Smith for the brutal beating of Alice.

The doctor decided to keep Alice in the hospital at least overnight to make sure she had not suffered internal injuries. The following morning Patrick went into town and picked Alice up returning her to the house.

\*\*\*\*\*\*\*\*\*

## CHAPTER 18

Every time I go to check on Fred I get a little thrill just seeing him. What the hells wrong with me? How could I dream of him holding me, making love to me and telling me how much he cared for me? DAMN!!

Fred no longer asks to be freed. He seems perfectly happy and I think I see desire in his face. It is probably just my hopeful thinking. When I bathe him, no longer needing to drug him he hardens up and leans into me, touching my face and lately my breast, giving me much pleasure. I've got to have him. I'm just afraid of what he may do if he could get his hands around my neck. Maybe he is just pretending, just hoping to get the chance to kill me…but then he could never hope to get out and with no one to bring him food and water, he would die as well.

Today as I undress him for his bath and change of clothes, my whole being is on fire. I want him desperately. I have questioned him and found he had gotten cured of the venereal disease he had given to me. Goodness but he is beautiful.

I leaned my breast against his face as his hands pulled at my buttons freeing my breast not encumbered by a bra. His lips covered my left breast as his hand massaged my right one. Soon his lips were caressing my entire body as I allowed my clothes to slip down to my ankles. I quickly pushed my clothing away with my foot and stood before him as naked as the day I was born. I can feel Fred's body vibrate as he moans and holds me. "My love, my love!" is all he says. I can no longer stand. I drop to the bed as Fred's naked body covered my body still nursing at my breast and rubbing me everywhere. "Let me baby. Please let me," he begged. I raised my arms to encircle his body and pushed my body closer to him. Waves of pleasure racked my body. I screamed and held him to me, never wanting to let him go. "I love you Gracie, I love you," he panted. This can't be. I have him imprisoned here. He no longer has his freedom to live as he pleases. He must be pretending just to get me to let him go. Fred continues to hold me and to kiss me until he is once again giving me pleasure, the like of which I have never known. All I can think of is more, please more.

It is six a.m. when I awake still in Fred's arms. He is still holding me, even in sleep. I try to slip out of his arms but I can't without waking him. "Fred, I must go," I whisper, but he holds me tighter.

"Again." he said. "Please again. Let me love you once more before you leave," he begged.

We made wonderful, sweet, tender love with a more complete fulfillment on every level.

It's a busy time on the plantation now and I can hardly contain myself from running back to Fred. All day long I have re-lived our night of passion and love. Yes love, real love. I am crazy for him. I must hurry through my duties so I can be with him again.

I took a folding card table and some board games along with some crossword puzzle books and I dragged a padded rocker down that passageway as well. With my basket full of good food, wine, cheese and an ice cream bar I finish today's supplies to Fred.

As soon as he saw me he reached his arms to me and I hurried into them. After kisses and love words I handed Fred the ice cream bar to eat before it melted. "Thank you but I'd rather taste on you," he said. We ate our fill and I showed him the card table and the rocker.

"Thanks baby, this bed does get uncomfortable to sit on with no back rest," he said.

"Is there anything else I can do for you?"

"Yes, lots. Give me lots of kisses. Tell me you love me a thousand times and prove it here in my arms."

As we undress each other I want to jump right on him and gobble him up. I want every square inch of him inside of me. I want his lips to nurse my breasts, to give me those tiny bites all over my body. I want to do the same to him. Again and again we make love never wanting to let go. too soon morning comes and we have to part. "Think of me while you are out," Fred says.

"You are all I ever think of."

Today I am going to try to get another chair through the passageway. I'm not sure I can because it is very heavy. I'll have to roll it end over end until I get it to where Fred lives. It is getting to be where it seems normal for Fred to be there and for me to sleep there in his arms. I can envision no life without him nor of having any change in circumstances. I like feeling he is mine to do with as I please. I can order him to do anything or I can order him to stop at any time.

Somehow that adds to the overall pleasures. If I wanted to I could beat him or make him follow me around on his knees for as far as the chain would reach. I can with hold food and water or I can with hold myself, which I certainly do not want to do. The more I order him around, the more he seems to love it as he begs, "Love me, let me love you, please, please." The more he begs the more sexually aroused we both become. He begs me to spank him with the ruler, which I do. Afterwards I kiss the welts and rub them with lotion. Now he is ready to deliver lovemaking as I have never even heard about. His stamina is amazing and mine is as well.

"Fred?" I asked, "If I let you go, will you have me arrested?"

"Please Gracie, don't let me go. I want to be right here with you, forever. I've never been so happy in my life. Women have always tagged around after me, doing for me. I didn't know then why I couldn't get overly excited over them, now I know. I must be dominated to be happy. All I ever want is to give you whatever pleasure I can in any way I can. Never, never let me go," he gasps as he holds my hands.

Everyone comments on happy I look and sound. "What's your secret?" the kitchen girls asked.

"Just good health, good living and realizing I have every possible thing I need to be happy I guess."

I went to the hair dresser where I had my hair styled and a little color added. My nails were getting raggedy as well so I also had them done. I bought myself some filmy diaphanous nighties and some silk pajamas for Fred in several colors, fine house slippers and a wrist watch for him also.

I'm taking special goodies tonight. It's our first anniversary and ends a year of the happiest memories of my lifetime.

I believe I must be what is called a dominatrix. I so enjoy controlling Fred and I'm so happy he loves for me to rule him. Tonight I'm taking a riding crop that I purchased into the dungeon with me. I can just feel the sting of the leather as I bring it down on Fred's back and buttocks. I can hardly wait. I picked up an eight by ten carpet from one of the empty apartments to put on the floor by Fred's bed. He has been working at leveling the dirt floor and placing planks that I have taken down there one at a time over the past year.

We now have a very nice love nest with every convenience except that the chemical toilet has to be emptied and the contents buried in that same space where Francious's grandfather emptied his chamber pot so many years ago. Now however I pour chemicals into the hole as well as in the chemical toilet. There is no foul odor at all now. I use the same chemical as motor homes use. It liquifies everything and it all soaks into the ground.

Fred no longer wears the chain when I am there but he insists I chain him when I am ready to leave. It is so wonderful that we match each other's needs so well.

As I come into Fred's line of sight I swish the riding crop through the air. His eyes are shining with anticipation.

"Get back," I bark at him. "You have been bad, very bad and now I must punish you!" I say shaking the crop at him.

"Yes my love. I have been a very bad boy. I deserve to be punished. Whip me! Whip me hard. I need it. I need it!" he cried as he yanked his clothes off. I could see he was already in a state of excitement. My clothes joined his clothes in a heap as I struck his back over and over, just hard enough to raise welts but not bring blood. By now he was wild reaching for me, crying out his love and need. "Now, now," he pleaded, "let me, oh let me!"

"No!" I screamed. "You may not have me. You are bad!" I said as I struck him several times more with him begging me to beat him harder. I really wanted to harm him badly. I needed to bite him hard and I feel as though I must tear at his flesh until his blood flows. I must not. I won't. I love him. Why do I feel this overpowering need to really hurt him. "Please don't let me do this terrible thing," I whispered.

Finally I am in control of myself and I kneel beside Fred's red skinned body. I kiss his stripes, his face, his chest while I say love words to him. Our lovemaking is the best it has ever been for me and Fred says for him as well. He is ecstatic, avowing his love for me, asking me to punish him some more, but I won't. I may not be able to stop.

I'm having misgivings about this dominatrix thing I have found myself to be. Why do I get such pleasure from inflicting pain upon the person I love? I must keep these feelings buried but how can I when Fred begs me to beat him? Sometimes I feel as though he wants to be bloodied or worse. What is this sickness? Where has it come from in me? I've had a great life, a wonderful family, no ill treatment, no broken homes or battered women in the family. I've never had to struggle for anything and I love my position in the family. Maybe I will go see Dr. Foley, but can I talk to him without telling him the facts. I absolutely cannot do that.

Dr. Foley listened to my tale about a friend. He told me my friend needs a psychiatrist and his personal feelings on this particular illness is to stay away from places where it is likely to inflame the need to an even higher plane.

I'm sure he knows I'm the friend, but I cannot take his advice. I must go to Fred often to calm my raging hormones that took so long to surface.

Family members gathered at Plantation House to celebrate Patrick's twenty seventh birthday. I hope to speak to him in private in the next few weeks. Patrick has proven himself a capable trustworthy person and so has Jack. With Hilda getting along in years I expect Jack will be chosen by Patrick to share the secrets and the running of the plantation for the next twenty or so years. Things are changing so rapidly in this world it is not a certainty Plantation House will continue to exist by the same standards. I can only hope that each generation produce people of character to keep the family in control of the whole plantation.

I have been putting everything in order in preparation for my trip to Paris. I have my passport up to date and my ticket purchased to Dallas, Texas where I may spend a few days before leaving for Paris. I have left my will and two sealed envelopes addressed to Patrick with pertinent information about or connected with Plantation House and the running thereof. My mind is much clearer now that I've decided upon a course of action.

Fred and I are still supremely happy. Fred no longer needs the chain but insists on wearing it. However I do leave the key to the cuff that encircles his ankle so he can remove it at any time. I've shown him the secret latch and how to get through the opening. We now spend a great deal of time in my quarters but we only make love below. Having a shower is a great treat for Fred. He spends quantity and quality time just letting the water soak his flesh. Sometimes at night we slip out of the house for fresh air and exercise. Life is wonderful, or could be if I could rid myself of these terrible urges to torture my darling Fred. I have prayed for help and I have discussed it with Fred, who is no help at all. The more I speak of what I want to do to him, the more excited he becomes.

I have gotten books from the library containing information on domination, sadism, and masochism. I've discovered there are tens of thousands of us in the world so now I don't feel so different as I did. Still I'd give everything I own to be rid of the forceful urges and for Fred to be less needy of punishment in order to experience full sexual gratification. it is as if there is no other reason to be, no reason to continue to breathe. I find myself fantasizing on having a room full of people to whip and bite hunks out of. I've got to do something or go crazy - crazier.

I'm like a maddened animal. The more sexually aroused I become the more I want to beat and tear the flesh right off of Fred's body. The more violent I become, the more Fred begs me to tear at him and he becomes more aroused and capable of long, enduring sexual sessions. often my darling is so sore he can hardly move with whip lashes and teeth marks all over his body. I hold him and rub salves and lotions all over his wounds as he whimpers and tells me how much he loves me and that he will be a good boy.

The days are passing with speed. Very soon now I will be on my way hopefully for a happier existence. My bags are packed and waiting by the door. I've made arrangements for a cab to pick me up. I've explained to everyone that this is the way I want it to be. I have spoken to Patrick and told him to take an envelope from the library in six months marked, open in private, if I have not returned by that date.

\*\*\*\*\*\*\*\*\*

# CHAPTER 19

"Patrick, where is that new man working today? I wanted to line him out for then next week on the restocking of the hay and grain storage enclosures," said Jack.

"I believe that Oscar is putting fuel into the tractor," I answered.

Since Gracie left I have not had enough free time to oversee the workings at the barn and still do all the tasks connected with Plantation House and it's staff. Gracie had suggested we dissolve Grover School for Girls. The income from the tuition fees is negligible to the problems of the running of the school.

Now I have to search for a replacement for Hilda as she wants to retire. None of our present kitchen help are capable of running the kitchen and the hiring and firing of all house staff. I have placed ads in the southern states papers for housekeeper/foreman for Plantation House. Perhaps I will find someone with experience in managing a large house and staff.

It's time to run the books before we send them to the accountants for filing I.R.S. taxes. Our income after expenses this year is considerable and will require a large sum to pay off the taxes. In the history of Plantation House there has never been a time since the plantation has been under cultivation and stocked animals that we have not made a good profit and each year it gets better. We keep up with all the modern planting practices and buy the best seeds and plants available.

Our stock is the best beef cattle anyplace. Our help is the most capable we can find. On our newest acquisition of a thousand acres plus buildings, we have hired a family that runs a dairy on that farm and truck farms fruits and vegetables for sale and for canning to supply all of the employees on the plantation with fresh and canned goods. The hogs have also been transferred to the new addition leaving room for new calf enclosures to protect them from predator animals as well as protection from the weather.

This is much more demanding than I envisioned it to be. It seems as though there is a new emergency every day. Someone gets ill, someone quits, someone has to be let go, someone refuses to wash windows and so on and on and on.

I have had a couple of responses to my advertisement for a new head person to run things. The references are being checked plus our personal investigator is doing a rundown on the applicants. It is so important to have quality people in charge of Plantation House. Our guarantee of only the very best is all important to maintain our reputation.

It has been three months and we have not heard anything from Gracie. She seemed so out of character for months before she left. It was as if something were hanging over her, something she could not rid herself of. Perhaps she will get around to writing or calling soon. Gracie has always been a little different than uncles Jonathan and Thomas, almost as if they were not brothers and sister. The boys lived normal lives, getting married and having children. Aunt Gracie left to live the life of a Bohemian artist for years. Even when she returned home she did not really mingle with the rest of the family. Oh she puts in appearances but somehow isn't there in spirit.

We have been scraping chipped paint and filling in any cracks on the house. It takes over two months just to get it covered in paint with three or four men working at it daily. Still the splendor of Plantation

House is incomparable. She stands like a beautiful goddess as if defiant to time and the elements and her style is as modern looking as the day it was built.

Today we replaced two tractors and a jeep. We believe that it is more cost effective to purchase new equipment every ten years than to spend time and money to keep older machinery working properly. The new silo is filled with silage and the barns are filled with grain and hay for outdoor feeding stations this coming winter.

I love watching the baby animals frolic, running, kicking up their heels and pouncing on one another. We no longer have the hogs here but baby pigs are my favorite animal of all. They look as though they are standing on tiptoe as they run squealing about.

I have finally located a person that may be able to fill Hilda's position. At least this is hopefully true. I still have to see her in person, however her resume sounds like what we need here to keep things humming and running smoothly.

"Hello Celia," I spoke as I held my hand out to welcome her. "Are you ready to go to work?"

"I am if I feel as I can fill the job and if you think I can do the job as you require it to be done," she replied.

Celia is a hefty well built woman of thirty eight, never married and no children. She has worked the better part of her life as housekeeper and companion to a widowed lady on a large plantation in Georgia that has recently passed away. She appears friendly and eager to please. I hope she can handle the job. I've really been plagued by female complaints. I do not necessarily like the book keeping and check writing, but I can tolerate it better than I can the constant complaints of women.

It is six months and two days since I last spoke to Gracie when she was about to leave for Paris after telling me, "If you do not hear from me in six months, I will be dead. Go then to the library and open the letter addressed to you, after reading it, destroy it. Do exactly as it says. I am so very sorry to leave this way. I have problems I cannot confide to anyone. They are shameful and I do not wish the family to be made aware of my personal life."

I retrieved the letter, sitting down to read it I have a foreboding feeling. I can't imagine what she could be so distraught about or what could be so shameful that she could not share it with at least one of us. I'm sure something could have been down to help her.

The letter reads, "My dear nephew. If you are reading this letter, I am I hope in a better place. Wait the seven years required by law to have a person declared dead. At that time read the second letter addressed to you, before my will is read and in private. It will explain many things that I am not ready to divulge at this time. If any of the monies in my safes are needed feel free to use it all if necessary. Take care of Plantation House and all of her secrets. My best, Gracie."

I'm no more aware of why Gracie left or why she assumed she would be dead by now. Why did she feel she would prefer to die alone or amongst strangers than surrounded by family. Also what secrets is she alluding to connected to Plantation House?

\*\*\*\*\*\*\*\*\*

# CHAPTER 20

The long black hearse is pulling out into the driveway taking my second son to the graveyard where all the habitants of Plantation House are interred a quarter of a mile just inside the gate that allows entrance into the grounds. I cannot view him being lowered into the ground and having dirt shoveled over him. I doubt I will be able to speak to anyone for sometime. His time was short and his death sudden from a fall off the back of a rearing horse that had been frightened by a snake. Jess was a son to be proud of. He was always laughing and never complained about chores he was expected to do. I have always expected Jess to be the one to take my place at Plantation House when I retire. I see him every place I look and remember his energy and the pranks he pulled on me and the rest of the family. I don't think I can ever eat another donut. They were Jess's favorite and he hit the kitchen smiling, hand out for a donut several times a day. "Dear God, hold my hand."

Darrell my first son is very quiet these days. He goes around doing the chores Jess usually had done after he finishes his own assigned jobs. I have never seen him cry, not a tear but I can tell his heart is broken and he misses Jess so much. He will soon be a teenager and the plans the two of them had to join the navy for at least one tour of duty is now a forgotten dream.

He says, "I'm no longer considering joining the navy. It just wouldn't be the same now."

I try to talk to him and the youngest son Timothy encouraging them to go on with their lives. We can never forget Jess even if we wanted to, which we don't, but he would want us to be happy. We must try to accept God's will. "Why would God make Jess die?" asked Timmy.

"God did not make Jess die. It was just his allotted time."

"Why did God allot that day for Jess to die?"

"I don't know Timmy. I've often tried to find the answers to such things. It is just the way of things."

"Well I don't like it and I think it is wrong to have good people die before they even get a chance to live," said Timmy.

"That's the way I think too," Darrell said. The tears finally came. He sobbed his heart out. "I miss Jess so much," he choked.

I held both my boys and tried to comfort them. My two baby daughters, ages one and three looked on sadly not understanding why we were all crying. I am so glad they are too young to hurt.

My wonderful wife is devastated. She has been in bed for days with a cold cloth over her eyes. The maid has taken over for her and Celia has fed and bathed the small ones each day and tucked them into bed at night.

Celia is a jewel. We are so fortunate to have found her. Since she took over in the kitchen they have gone back to cooking in pots and pans. They roast and bake in the stove ovens not in micro waves. Our six micro waves have been stored in the basement except for the very large one for the kitchen help to use for themselves if they care to. also micro waves are great to reheat food if something should delay the meals but food cooked in them just does not taste as good as food cooked the conventional way.

The years are passing. Darrell is in the navy. Timmy is in his last year of school here where tutors have taught all the children.

Timmy is the one that wishes to stay on the plantation and eventually take over my duties. I would never have believed Tim would be the one who loves ranching and every phase of running the place. He has worked beside his cousin who tends to all the cattle diseases. Tim isn't going to veterinarian school. He says, "There ain't nuthin I ain't dealt with where a cow, pig, horse and even chickens are concerned for the past five years. If that won't do it, too bad," Tim boasted. I agree, he has learned the trade through hands on experience and he has read every book on what a vet does for hundreds of ailments animals may suffer.

This is the anniversary of Gracie's leaving. I often think of her and wonder whatever happened to her that caused her to leave and how she knew she would be dead in six months.

Jack's eldest is going into the marines for one tour he says, "Then I am coming home, getting married and have a house full of kids. They are all going to love it here and fight for the right to live our their lives, right here."

Jack and I look at each other, both of us thinking, "Yeah!"

I love every year better and more than I did the last year. I love just lying on a horse blanket gazing at the acres and acres of beautiful land. The cattle are fat and healthy, I'm in paradise. I couldn't ask for heaven to be any better except for the loss of Jess and the mystery

of Gracie. I am a happy man. There is nothing on God's green earth

that could be any better in my opinion.


\*\*\*\*\*\*\*\*\*

# CHAPTER 21

Tomorrow we gather to hear Gracie's will and I will read the letter which I hope gives some answers to the life and death of Gracie.

I take the letter in hand, a trembling hand to read. I have such a dread to see the contents. The front of the envelope says, "Read in private."

The will is a standard will with gifts to some of the family but most of her per personal wealth is to go back into the fund to keep Plantation House in perfect repair for as long as a member of our family survives. No mention as to the reason for her departure.

The letter states; "Patrick, you will understand why I wanted you to wait the seven years when I could be declared legally dead to read this letter and to visit the secret passage I shall tell you about. I want you to know that I am ashamed and I really did try to overcome my ugly urges, but I could not.

I have left journals as did Francious's grandfather. Inside his hand printed books you will find many answers and in my journal you will find many more answers you must not reveal to the rest of the family. They would only hurt and shame the rest of the family. You must keep secret, the passageway that leads to the dungeon until it is time to relinquish the care and secrets to a most trusted member of the family.

I have drawn you a map that shows the three secret openings. Do not leave this map anywhere that someone may accidently stumble upon it.

When you go into the dungeon you will find a large yellow jacketed journal that will explain all that you will see."

I took the map and went into Gracie's now empty quarters. Finding the secret latch I entered the passageway where I flicked on the light switch that was just inside the opening. Making my way forward I come upon an opening where furniture, carpets, paintings, trunks and other varied boxes and a bed stood. A bed sheet that was covered with copious amounts of dried blood lay atop what looked like the body of a man and a woman judging by the hair and the size of the feet. One large skeletal foot bore what looked like an ankle bracelet about four inches wide. There was no odor. Seven years had decayed what rats and other varmints had not done away with. My

God, this must be Gracie, but who is the man and how did he get here? How did Gracie get back here from Paris? Why?? I quickly pick up the yellow journal that topped several other journals, beginning to read.

"Patrick, I did not go to Paris or any place else. I simply returned after everyone was asleep and slipped back into this place. You will find journals telling who this is with me and my hideous crime, for when you read this I will have long ago killed my lover and myself. We were both sick people who fell in love and filled a need for each other.

My illness is abhorrent, so is his. We cannot survive apart and I cannot control my need to injure him as he cries out for me to do more harm to him. The more I beat and tear hunks out of him the higher his gratification and mine as well. After my darling is dead I'll drink the dissolved sleeping pills I've saved up from Dr. Foley's prescriptions as well as hand full of muscle relaxing tablets I've saved up and I'll go to sleep, never to wake again.

Now you can see why I had to do what I did to protect the family and Plantation House. Please forgive me and think kindly of me if you can. Love Gracie.

P.S. As I beat and tore hunks from my darling's flesh he begged for more. I tore his eyes from their sockets and slashed his face with his straight razor as he screamed in ecstasy. There are no words to describe the height of my sexual gratification. May God forgive me. G."

What am I going to do? How can I live knowing of this gruesome slaughter. However, wouldn't it be worse to have everyone know and discuss it forever more. "Help me to know what to do," I prayed.

Life goes on much the same here as it has since 1779. The secrets that Plantation House hold are inviolate. I have kept the secrets and will one day give over the map to Timmy. I hope he also will keep the secrets of Plantation House until the next master takes over.

\*\*\*\*\*\*\*\*\*

**{Fini}**

# ABOUT THE AUTHOR

Born in Oklahoma, 12/23/25, she is the eldest of eight children. She married at age fourteen to get away from home.

A first daughter was born fifteen months later followed by two more daughters by nineteen years of age. One son Billy Earl, was born 3/12/49. He is now deceased.

At age 75 Ms. Neeley decided to try her hand at writing. Secrets of Plantation House being one of eight novels.

www.ingramcontent.com/pod-product-compliance
Lightning Source LLC
Chambersburg PA
CBHW022248290526
45785CB00015B/399